DEDICATION

I dedicate this book to my late father, Miguel Angel Espinosa,
who trusted me in successfully taking care of his prostate
naturally till the very end. Te quiero y te extraño, Papi.

THRIVE DON'T ONLY SURVIVE

THRIVE DON'T ONLY SURVIVE

DR.GEO'S GUIDE TO LIVING YOUR BEST LIFE BEFORE & AFTER PROSTATE CANCER

IMPLEMENT THE SCIENCE OF THE CAPLESS METHOD

Dr. Geo Espinosa N.D., L.Ac

This book is intended to supplement, not replace, the advice of a trained health professional. If you know or think you have a health problem, you should consult with a health professional. The author and publisher specifically disclaim any liability, loss, or risk, personal or otherwise, that is incurred as a consequence, directly or indirectly, of the use and application of any contents of this book.

ISBN-13: 9781517287825
ISBN-10: 1517287820
Library of Congress Control Number: 2015914891
Createspace Independent Publishing Platform
North Charleston, South Carolina

Thank you for your support of the author's rights.

Riverdale Publisher
PO Box 167
Bronx, New York 10471

DISCLAMER

Although the author and publisher have made every effort to ensure that the information in this book was correct at press time, the author and publisher do not assume and hereby disclaim any liability to any party for any loss, damage, or disruption caused by errors or omissions, whether such errors or omissions result from negligence, accident, or any other cause.

This book is not intended as a substitute for the medical advice of physicians. The reader should regularly consult a physician in matters relating to his/her health and particularly with respect to any symptoms that may require diagnosis or medical attention.

TABLE OF CONTENTS

FOREWORD

I HAVE PERSONALLY known Dr. Geo Espinosa for many years. As the Director of the Holistic Center at Columbia University, I hired Dr. Geo to evaluate and see the patients diagnosed with prostate cancer and offer advice nutritionally as well as improve their quality of life. In many cases, that also meant reducing their stress load and dealing with the anxiety of being told that you have prostate cancer. What impressed me most about Dr. Geo was he was empathic approach to each and every man and his tireless dedication to patients, employing many of the tools that he learned as an naturopathic physician.

In his first book, "Thrive -Don't Only Survive" he is able to communicate the knowledge that he has learned through his countless hours of research and consulting on thousands of men and their spouses. His humble approach with patients is inspiring, and the messages within each chapter are clear and ring throughout the book.

As part of his holistic "big picture" approach (which he has coined the CaPLESS method) to prostate cancer, Dr. Espinosa offers a clear, easy-to-follow regimen of herbs and vitamins as well as stress reduction techniques and exercises to follow. His diet, one that is low in saturated fats (meats, dairy, butter) and rich in olive oil, flaxseeds and flax oil and other sources of omega-3 and omega-6 fatty acids (salmon, sardines, cod) as well as anti-oxidant-rich organic fruits and vegetables (particularly blueberries and members of the crucifer family) and fermented soy-based foods (tempeh and miso) is detailed.

Although his book deals with prostate cancer, it is likely that the diet and integrative approach that he embraces could apply to many cancers that men and women face in 2015. I applaud him for his continued efforts in giving men wonderful advice for healthy living and for the energy and dedication that he gave for writing this wonderful book.

Dr. Aaron Katz, MD
Winthrop University Hospital,
Department of Urology,
Chairman

INTRODUCTION

This journey of a thousand miles begins with a single step.

—LAO TZU

YOU HAVE PROSTATE cancer!

Few phrases have the power to induce more emotion. Few words can provoke so much uncertainty, confusion, and fear like "cancer." After the initial diagnosis, a series of thoughts bounces around in a man's head: How bad is it? How long do I have to live? What treatments are available to me? Will the treatment ruin my quality of life? Will I be able to see my kids and grandchildren grow?

Stop and take a moment.

Having seen thousands of patients with prostate cancer at my New York clinic, I can tell you that every man faced with this situation asks himself similar questions and confronts the same anxieties. You are not alone.

More than 2.5 million men in the United States and more than 1 billion in the world live with prostate cancer. Even more concerning—about 40 percent of prostate cancer returns after treatment with surgery or radiation. Holy crap!

So after you go through the stress, pain, and urinary and sexual side effects of initial treatment, you have the chance of it returning? Yup. And even worse off are men who refuse to change their lifestyle habits after treatment, naively thinking they are cancer-free. Prostate cancer is a red flag that your body is "cancering," not just your prostate. After all, your prostate is connected to the rest of your body, so you have to ask yourself: Where else am I harboring cancer cells that I don't know about yet? If you have or had prostate cancer, then you must take immediate action to lower your risk of prostate cancer recurrence and reduce your chances of developing cancer at another location.

This is why the CaPLESS Method is so important. You see, prostate cancer is a life-changing situation for you, I know. But not in the way you think. Prostate cancer is likely not a death sentence since fewer than 12 percent of men die from it after diagnosis. Odds are something else will get you long before your prostate cancer does. So your life is far from over. In fact, it is only beginning.

Your diagnosis is an opportunity to ask yourself: Do you want to be a survivor—or a thriver? Do you want to use this new chapter of your life to be stronger and increase your life expectancy? Or do you want to remain stuck in your old ways and habits? In no part of this program do I exaggerate. There are no smoke and mirrors here. Prostate cancer is your opportunity to live your best life yet.

Who were you before your prostate cancer? Did you:

- Eat a lot of processed foods and empty calories?
- Have a big gut?
- Rarely, if ever, move on a regular basis?
- Exist under a constant cloud of work and everyday stress?

How would you like to change these answers and rapidly rid your body of cancer-causing toxins, have more energy, slim down, and in the process help to better create a cancer-hostile environment in your body?

It is possible. And I will show you how.

Before we continue, I'd like to thank you for trusting me to take you through the journey of rebuilding, reclaiming, and renewing your health. I know there are a lot of books and material on the Internet competing for your attention, claiming the next natural cure for cancer.

I feel privileged to enter this relationship with you through this book. Also, congratulations to you for choosing to take the "bull by the horns" with determination and courage as you move toward a better you. I know it hasn't been easy, but today is a new beginning.

For over a decade, I have operated as a naturopathic urology doctor, counseling thousands of patients with prostate cancer in New York City, first at Holistic Urology Center at Columbia University Medical Center and now as director of the Integrative Urology Center at New York University's Langone Medical Center.

But I did not stop there. I know there is not only one way of doing things and what works for one person may not work for another. This is why I have also spent countless hours researching which natural strategies have the greatest impact on prostate cancer—from entire diet plans to individual foods to fitness routines to supplements to lifestyle choices. You name it, and I have probably researched it.

Along the way, I have also discovered what doesn't work. It turns out many patients I see are on the wrong diets and taking supplements that worsen their cancer risk. While the Internet can be a useful resource, it's also filled with false information and dangerous promises.

The result from my personal clinical experience, observations, and scientific research is a systematic lifestyle plan I call the CaPLESS Method. It provides what I have found to be the best tools for men to reclaim what I believe is their right—their health.

A prostate cancer diagnosis offers the amazing opportunity to take immediate action—reevaluate your life, figure out what's important and what isn't, rekindle important relationships, love more, and stress less. With the CaPLESS Method, you will move beyond being a prostate cancer survivor to becoming a vibrant prostate cancer thriver.

I detest the word "survivor"—especially when preceded by "cancer." The words you speak to yourself create a corresponding emotion. Remember the feeling when your physician informed you that your biopsy came up positive for prostate cancer? Your stomach tightened. You probably experienced chills.

"Survivor" implies that you are just making it. You are hanging in there, barely. The words you use to describe your life experiences are connected in the part of the brain called the hypothalamus. The hypothalamus controls virtually all of the different chemicals produced in your body. Disempowering words can be stressful—producing hormones and neurotransmitters that weaken your body.

That's what the word "cancer" does to you when it sneaks into your brain. "Survivor," while a better word, is still not great. Because simply surviving is not enough. The ultimate goal is to live your *best* life—in other words, to "thrive." How about "CaPLESS thriver"? "CaP" is an abbreviation of "carcinoma of the prostate," but the actual words have more meaning than abbreviations. The impact of words on health has been studied by many scientists. So the term we will use to describe a better you will be "CaPLESS thriver."

THE CAPLESS METHOD: THRIVE, DON'T ONLY SURVIVE

CaPLESS stands for: CaP (carcinoma of the prostate)—medical jargon that stands for "prostate cancer"—"L" is for "lifestyle," "E" is for "exercise," "S" is for sleep (and stress) and the last "S" is for "supplementation." The CaPLESS Method is a science-based intervention program on the lifestyle and behavior routines that will keep you living your best life from this day forward.

You may wonder, "If the concepts of the CaPLESS Method work so well, why hasn't my doctor told me about them?" I'm asked this question at least once a day.

If you expect your conventional physician to make naturopathic/lifestyle recommendations, you're likely to be disappointed. Conventional physicians are passionate about bringing a cure to patients, but many are not trained in nutritional or naturopathic interventions—only in drug and surgical treatments.

While aggressive treatments are sometimes necessary, they don't build health. The CaPLESS Method is about building the health of your whole body to create an inhospitable environment for cancer—not simply to treat prostate cancer. I strongly believe that treating prostate cancer with surgery, radiation, or any of a dozen or so other therapies, without the patient applying a lifestyle approach like the CaPLESS Method, falls short. After all, prostate cancer is not a local problem, it's a systemic one.

I suspect that this is why biochemical relapse occurs more than 40 percent of the time after treatments that are intended to cure. You have to treat the host—you. No one bothers to treat "Mr. Jones," the person, where the cancer resides. And yet, prostate cancer is not an isolated entity. It is part of someone's body. Without treating the person, the biological soil of the prostate cancer, a long-term cure and optimal wellness are almost impossible.

Urologists and oncologists focus on perfecting their skills in eradicating cancer, which of course is important, but often offers little support for you, the patient, when you leave the doctor's office. You are sort of left high and dry after treatment.

This is why you need to take charge and actively participate in your road to wellness. You are the one living with prostate cancer, so with the right strategy, it is up to you to do something about it.

This book is not about what treatment options you should choose, or which are necessarily best. That's a conversation between you and your physician. This book does not replace the proper advice from him or her.

Instead, this book is about you—a man confronting his prostate cancer—and how to embrace a new means of living. In the following pages, you will learn how you can create a structured and more natural lifestyle. One that is based on natural medicine and real science. One that not only will help you manage your prostate cancer, but will perhaps become an integral part of reversing your disease, all while helping you to live healthier than ever before.

FIVE STAGE APPROACH TO GOING CAPLESS

First, I will explain why you have prostate cancer, or why it returned after treatment, how the common medical treatments work, and how to navigate through the false information and Internet hype.

Next I will explore in detail how each of the five main pillars of the CaPLESS Method operates—**Eating, Movement, Supplementation, Stress Management** and **Sleep.**

Then, I will show you how to begin implementing the program into your life with a 21-Day Reset, which jump-starts your body to begin healing, and help you to embrace a more positive mind-set and establish the CaPLESS Method as a way of life.

Lastly, I will offer insight into how to include the CaPLESS Method in the treatment option you choose for your prostate cancer, and how to the make the program sustainable for the long haul. And along the way, you will also hear stories from men just like you and their partners who have embraced the CaPLESS Method and how it has changed their lives.

It doesn't matter who you are—whether you are 50, recently diagnosed with advanced prostate cancer, and reviewing your options, or if you have prostate cancer recurrence, or if you're somewhere in-between. The CaPLESS Method can work for you.

I also understand that prostate cancer is not just about you. Your diagnosis affects everyone in your life, but especially your significant other. The partner in your life needs to be involved with your health (and trust me, he or she wants to).

Prostate cancer is rarely a solo journey, which is why another key aspect of the CaPLESS Method is what I call, "Note to Life Partner," where I speak straight to the life partner of a man with prostate cancer. I offer suggestions on how they can help him during all phases of the CM, including when to offer advice, support, or just be there for him. Plus this gives a couple an opportunity to embrace a new way of living—together.

What life partners will also discover is that they too can benefit from the CaPLESS Method. Eating better, adopting more movement, getting adequate sleep, and controlling stress is good for everyone's health and well-being and can perhaps help them stave off cancer and other illnesses, as well.

Yes, you have battled prostate cancer, but do you want to just stay alive—or live your best life possible? One filled with vitality, strength and longevity—a productive life shared with those you love. Do you want to just survive—or thrive?

CHAPTER 1

YOU HAVE PROSTATE CANCER—NOW WHAT?

Let me not die while I am still alive.

—*Jewish Prayer*

I HAVE NOTICED many men tune out the specifics of their diagnosis and treatment options once they hear the word "cancer" come out of their physician's mouth. Everything else that follows becomes sort of white noise.

Once you snap out of it, both you and your partner need to focus on how to make the best treatment choices. The more you educate yourself about prostate cancer, what it means, and the various available treatment options, the more confidence you will build. Embrace your new situation and you can begin to make positive changes that will improve your health.

No two men are alike and neither is their disease. Some may have early detection while others may discover it when it has progressed further. Some may be in their 40s or 50s while others are in their 70s. Someone may be pursuing aggressive treatment while another has adopted a wait-and-see approach, also known as active surveillance.

No matter where you are on the diagnosis and treatment spectrum, it is important to fully understand your situation, how your diagnosis was made, and your various treatment options (even if you have already chosen one).

The CaPLESS Method does not replace your current prostate cancer treatment. But it does complement it and strengthen the management of your condition and can be implemented into whichever path you choose.

In many ways, the CaPLESS Method will empower you and make the journey of treatment more tolerable, less stressful, and may even improve your outcome.

YOUR PROSTATE: A CLOSER LOOK

Let's take a step back and look at the source of your cancer. What is the prostate and why does it cause so much trouble?

When healthy, this gland is about the size and shape of a walnut and weighs about 20 to 30 grams. It lies just below the bladder, wrapped doughnut-like around a thin tube called the urethra that delivers urine and semen out through the penis. The prostate is composed of glandular tissue and muscle. It is divided into three lobes and surrounded by an outer casing called the prostatic capsule.

The prostate is a crucial gland in your sexual and reproductive system. Its main function is to produce most of the fluid in semen, the most important being a liquid protein called prostate-specific antigen, which you know as PSA. The job of PSA is to liquefy and protect semen on its way through the uterus to the female egg. PSA also serves as the controversial basis of PSA tests for cancer screening.

Unfortunately, the prostate's design is the root of many problems in aging men. As the calendar years add up, it begins to slowly grow. That's just the way it is. When enlarged or diseased, it squeezes the urethra like a kink in a garden hose, which blocks the flow of urine. If urine is blocked for too long, it can back up into the bladder and not empty fully. Left untreated, this blockage can permanently damage the bladder and eventually the kidneys.

The prostate's precarious placement also complicates treatment for both benign prostatic growth and cancer. Because the prostate is intertwined with so many crucial organs, nerves, and other important structures, it is difficult to remove or treat without causing damage to nearby tissues. Thus, treatment carries a risk of undesired side effects, such as impotence and incontinence.

Many older men mistake prostate cancer symptoms for normal signs of aging.

Early diagnosis is crucial, so do not ignore these warning flags:

- dribbling urine
- trouble urinating or an inability to urinate
- frequent urge to urinate
- burning or painful urination
- blood in the urine or semen
- painful ejaculation
- difficulty having an erection
- frequent pain in the lower back, hips or upper thighs

Every man over 50 should get screened for prostate cancer, especially if they experience any of these classic warning signs. If there is a strong family prostate cancer or breast cancer (even in females) medical history, I would recommend prostate cancer screening starting at 40 years old.

Keep in mind that the only way to know for certain if you have prostate cancer is with a biopsy, where samples of prostate cancer are extracted and analyzed in a lab. I say this because many men who see me at the clinic want a diagnosis without a biopsy. While some blood tests, imagings, and techniques are available for screening, a biopsy is still the gold standard for prostate cancer diagnosis. However, you can paint a picture of your current prostate health status before deciding to move to the more serious action of a biopsy. This begins with the iconic PSA test, which has been the standard starting point of diagnosis since the late 1980s, but has recently come under fire.

PSA TESTS

There are a many gray areas in understanding prostate cancer, and PSA is one of them. The prostate normally secretes a small amount of PSA into the blood. Enlargement, inflammation, and cancer allow more PSA than normal to enter the bloodstream. Some research suggests that even constipation could cause a PSA increase. The test measures the amount of PSA in your blood in nanograms (one-billionth of a gram) per milliliter (one-thousandth of a liter).

Traditionally, a PSA result of less than 4.0 ng/mL is considered normal. Your risk of prostate cancer increases as the number rises. Men over 50 have a 20 to 30 percent chance of having prostate cancer if their PSA level is between 4.1 and 10. If your PSA level is higher than 10, the possibility of cancer increases to 42 to 64 percent. When PSA is higher than 20, 80 percent of men are diagnosed with the disease. (Partin et al. 1994)

Sounds simple, but PSA tests can be flawed. It is not a 100-percent-accurate indicator of cancer risk. It is possible to have a PSA of less than 4 and still have cancer, or have a PSA of 15 and be cancer-free. You can also have false-positives where your PSA levels are artificially higher. This can be due to any of the following:

- You may have an unusually large prostate, which is non-cancerous, but produces more PSA simply because of its larger size.
- You may suffer from a prostate infection called prostatitis.
- You may have a urinary tract infection.
- You may have had sex within 48 hours before the test.

Another reason PSA has been criticized lately is that the results often set off an unnecessary chain reaction of expensive treatment. For instance, a man may have a PSA between 4.0 and 10, which statistically increases his risk of prostate cancer. It doesn't mean he *has* cancer, or will even get it. It only means he has a greater risk of developing prostate cancer.

Many men ignore the might and maybe. They hear these numbers and immediately want to take action, which can lead them down a long, somewhat painful, stressful, and expensive path of biopsy, surgery, radiation, and/or drug therapy, which can wreak havoc on their quality of life.

And in the end, it may not change how long they live. Always keep this in mind: You have a greater chance of dying from something other than prostate cancer. Yes, prostate cancer can be deadly, but remember, heart disease is still the number one killer of men worldwide. This is why so many in the medical field believe less emphasis should be placed on the PSA test.

Still, PSA tests do provide a valuable service, and are a good gauge of current risk—at least for now. But they should not be the only basis for any decision you make regarding treatment and long-term management. This is why it is often recommended that you pair your PSA results with other tests that can provide a clearer understanding of your current prostate health. These tests include the Prostate Cancer Antigen 3 (PCA 3), PSA Velocity (PSAV), PSA Density (PSAD), and Free PSA. Also, MRI imaging is more sophisticated and more reliable in detecting tumors of the prostate than ultrasounds.

Here is a look at each:

Prostate Cancer Antigen 3 (PCA 3)
PCA 3 is a genetic molecule found in a urine test to determine if prostate cancer is present. It is more specific to prostate cancer than PSA; however, studies have been conflicted in showing grade or stage of prostate cancer. For instance, a result higher than 35 means you may have prostate cancer, but it does not indicate whether it is low grade (and likely insignificant) or aggressive (and very significant).

PSA Velocity (PSAV)
PSAV is another tool to determine if aggressive screening for prostate cancer is appropriate. PSAV measures the significance of PSA changes over time. So, if your PSA today is a 2.0 and then in six months it's 4.0, your PSAV score is 2.0 over a six-month period. PSAV can also be used to determine if a biopsy should be considered as part of your prostate cancer screening. A PSAV of more than 2.0 in a year has been associated with a higher probability of cancer.

PSA Density (PSAD) is a measure of the amount of PSA relative to the overall prostate size in cubic centimeters as determined by ultrasound or MRI volume. PSAD is calculated by dividing the PSA number by the size of the prostate found in the ultrasound or MRI report. A high PSA density means that a relatively small size prostate is making a lot of PSA, a low PSA density means that a large size prostate is making relatively little PSA. A higher PSAD of more than 0.15 means a higher likelihood you have prostate cancer. Again, like PSA, you can have high value (more than 0.15) and not have prostate cancer. Also, as with PCA 3, PSAD does not tell the difference between aggressive and non-aggressive cancer. Some research argues that PSAD is more significant than PSA and Gleason score in determining aggressive prostate cancer. (Sfoungaristos & Perimenis, 2012)

Percent Free PSA. This test analyzes how much free PSA is traveling in the blood and how much of that is bound to a companion protein. If more than 25 percent of the PSA is free, chances are a noncancerous, but enlarged, prostate is producing it. If free PSA is lower than 15 to 25 percent, it is more likely that cancer is the cause. (Lee et al. 2015)

BIOPSY: RANDOM VS. TARGETED

If you do need a biopsy, which kind should you consider? Biopsies can be done in a doctor's office in about 10 minutes. There are two types: random and targeted. Random biopsies are performed with a process called a transrectal ultrasound (TRUS) guided biopsy. A physician, typically a urologist, inserts a probe in the rectum while identifying the prostate area of interest on a monitor. Then a thin needle is shot through the rectal tissue in a fraction of a second, to take small random samples of prostate tissue, called a core. The number of cores can vary, but the average is around 12.

Targeted biopsies, also known as MRI – ultrasound fusion biopsy are done with a TRUS along with the application of MRI and ultrasound images in order to target specific prostate tissue that appears suspicious. If a prostate biopsy is required and a targeted biopsy is accessible to you, then that's what you should choose.

Advantages of a targeted prostate biopsy compared to random biopsy include:

1. Lesser chance of finding indolent, non-life-threatening tumor (as indicated by a Gleason score of 6 or less).
2. Improved opportunity of finding aggressive tumors that may be deadly.
3. Excessive biopsies are avoided by finding tumors the first time.

Random needle TRUS biopsy is still the most popular method of prostate cancer diagnosis, but it has many problems. Aggressive cancers are often missed, harmless tumors are often found, excess biopsies are performed when PSA continues to rise, and sometimes a higher than usual amount of samples are taken (more than 20), which increases the risk of infection and erectile dysfunction. This is why I predict that random biopsies will be completely replaced by target biopsies within the next 5 to 10 years.

After a prostate biopsy of any type, tissue samples are sent to a pathologist for analysis under a microscope. The pathologist compiles a report that outlines the presence of cancer cells and the cancer's aggressiveness, which your doctor will explain to you.

Either biopsy will raise the risk of potential infection and cause some discomfort, but not serious pain. Your doctor will prescribe an antibiotic to take one day before and a few days after the procedure to avoid infection. You may experience a little soreness for about two weeks afterward, and you may notice blood in your urine or semen for a few weeks. Temporary erectile dysfunction after prostate biopsy has also been reported in some studies. (Murray et al. 2015)

Many patients ask me if it's possible to determine if they have prostate cancer without a biopsy. While it is true MRI images continuously improve, and other biomarkers like PCA 3 help with diagnosing prostate cancer, *a biopsy is still the only way any physician can conclusively make a diagnosis of prostate cancer.*

Yes, I know it doesn't sound pleasant, but a prostate biopsy is the gold standard for diagnosis, and no physician will be able to make a definite diagnosis without it.

That said, I strongly suggest you have at least two pathologists review your biopsy findings. Grading of prostate tissue is done visually, posing a risk of subjectivity and grading error. For this reason, Gleason scores (which I will address in the next section) can sometimes vary between pathologists. Additional biopsy readings can cost between $100 and $500 depending on the lab.

However, most insurance companies in the United States will cover this expense. Also, make sure to ask for your own records and to share them with all doctors on your health team.

THE GLEASON SCORE

Your biopsy is given a Gleason score. The Gleason score was developed by a pathologist named Dr. Donald Gleason in 1966 to measure the probability of aggressive prostate cancer. It is based on a scale of one to five, with one being the least aggressive cancer and five the most aggressive. The pathologist gives a score to two tumors and adds them up (i.e., 3+4, 4+3, etc.) to get your Gleason score. This final number ranges from 2 to 10: 2 to 4 (normal); 5 to 7 (less aggressive but still an intermediate risk); 8 to 10 (most aggressive and most serious).

The Gleason score is important because it can help predict the future course of your cancer, even if it has been caught early and does not yet appear to be serious. Your doctor will consider your Gleason score, along with the stage of your cancer, to help determine the best treatments for you. In general, the higher your stage of cancer, the bigger the threat to your life and the more aggressive treatment you may need.

Here are the main details of the biopsy report and what they mean:

- Tissue sample location: his can help your physician determine the best treatment method as some options are not ideal for tumors in hard to reach areas

- The percentage of the core that contains cancer (which could be expressed in mm of cancer size): this tells how much cancer is in each core and can help predict the cancer prognosis and course of treatment
- An indication of the Gleason grades and the percent for each grade
- An indication of any cancer found in nerves close to the prostate called the perineural invasion: this also can help with determining prognosis and best course of treatment
- Presence of HGPIN (High Grade Prostatic Intra-epithelial Neoplasia) or ASAP (Atypical Small Acinar Proliferation): this indicates cells that are abnormal, but not quite cancerous, or premalignant cells that often turn into cancer about 30 percent of the time. Patients with ASAP or HGPIN cells are monitored closely by their urologist since about 50 percent of repeat biopsies show cancer in this group of patients.
- An indication of any inflammation or prostatitis, which is a non-cancerous outcome and not precancerous

MULTIPARAMETRIC MAGNETIC RESONANCE IMAGING (MPMRI)

Multiparametric magnetic resonance imaging (mpMRI) is currently the most promising, noninvasive technique imaging test. It may be able to locate potentially deadly cancer while avoiding low-grade, harmless tumors, thus preventing unnecessary treatment. Multi-parametric means the performance of three scans sequentially during a single visit to the imaging center. The three scans are:

1. T2-weighted imaging: this allows for the best assessment of the prostate morphology, size, margins, and internal structures with easy differentiation between the prostate's various sections.
2. Diffusion-weighted imaging: this details the tissue microstructure and generates an apparent diffusion coefficient (ADC), which helps to determine the aggressiveness of a lesion if one is seen.

3. Dynamic contrast-enhanced imaging: this detects areas of increased vascularity to better detail any suspect lesions.

A radiologist reads the information from the three scans and compiles a report. Findings are then summarized in an overall impression, which falls into one of five categories:

1=clinically significant disease is highly unlikely to be present
2=clinically significant disease is unlikely to be present
3=clinically significant disease is equivocal
4=clinically significant disease is likely to be present
5=clinically significant disease is highly likely

For men treated with radiation, mpMRI can detect recurrence of prostate cancer with reasonable sensitivity compared with a biopsy.

GENOMIC TESTING
You and your physician want an answer to a very important question: Do you have the type of prostate cancer that can progress and eventually kill you or do you have the indolent type that will never grow, spread and lead to an early death?

Unfortunately, a biopsy alone can't always answer this question.

Prostate cancer and medicine in general involve probabilities like any other sector in life. As I mentioned earlier, random biopsies often fail to identify potentially deadly tumors. And while the "shoot-and-miss" component of the process has been greatly reduced by targeted biopsies, this method is not totally perfect, either.

Testing can further reduce your chances of missing an aggressive cancer that can be cured successfully if found early. And it can help you make an informed decision as to the best treatment process (such as deciding if an aggressive, mainstream approach is necessary at all).

There are three labs that offer Genomic Testing: Decipher® from GenomeDx (San Diego, CA), Onco*type*® from Genomic Health (Redwood City, CA) and Prolaris® from Myriad Genetics (Salt Lake City, UT).

Here's a quick summary of the difference:

Company	Name of Test	When is it performed?	What is analyzed?	What it tells you	What is the benefit?
GenomeDx	Decipher®	After surgical prostate removal	The prostate gland	Risk of cancer spread in 5 yrs or in 3 yrs after PSA recurrence	Tells you if additional salvage therapy needed
Genomic Health	Onco*type*®	After biopsy	Prostate tissue from biopsy	A genomic prostate score (GPS) showing the likelihood of having more aggressive cancer than the biopsy reports	Tells you if Active Surveillance is an option or if immediate treatment is required
Myriad Genetics	Prolaris®	After biopsy or surgical removal of the prostate	Prostate tissue from biopsy or prostate gland	Predicts 10-year survival with conservative management or chances of biochemical recurrence	Tells you if Active Surveillance is an option (after biopsy) or if immediate treatment is required (after prostatectomy)
MDx Health	Confirm-MDx®	After a prostate biopsy	It detects an epigenetic field based on DNA methylation	If there is a "halo effect" only present in cancer lesions from a biopsy	It confirms if a negative biopsy is truly negative or if there is hidden cancer not found by the biopsy

In the end, genomic testing helps you and your physician make a more informed decision as to what the next steps are in your journey toward a cancer-free life.

How do you talk to the newly diagnosed?

By David Guinther

There is no more potent a reminder of how fragile and fleeting life is than being diagnosed with cancer.

You may have family or friends who have been affected by cancer. As such, you may think that you understand what they are going through and how best to support and help them.

You don't.

Unless you have had the words "you have cancer" directed at you, you have no idea.

And I know this firsthand. I thought I understood, but apparently mortality is nothing more than an abstract concept until it is not.

Here are three suggestions on how best to talk to and help a loved one who is newly diagnosed with prostate or another form of cancer.

1. Appreciate the disorientation.

When I was diagnosed, I felt an immediate and deep sense of loss. Not just of my health, but of what I had envisioned as my shared future. Recognition of loss of control is profound. I lacked answers not just for myself, but also for all those for whom I needed to be strong. My initial goal was to try to make sense of it all.

And this takes time. So give your loved one time to live with and make sense of his new reality.

2. Don't try to fix it.

You cannot fix this problem for him. It is going to take time to properly assess and profile the disease prior to choosing the best course of treatment. Knowing the anxiety that uncertainty causes, please do not add to it by asking for answers or decisions on your timetable. This is his life, and he is seeking the best possible solution to a new and complex problem. He also wants answers, and the best possible outcome. So respect that.

3. Give him what he needs.

Offer patience, understanding, and unlimited support. Simply let him know that he matters to you, that you are thinking about him, and that you are here to help. He just needs to ask. He neither needs nor wants a pep talk, particularly one that references keeping a positive mental attitude.. He is already highly motivated to rebuild his health and reclaim his future.

If you simply cannot help yourself, limit your pep talk to encouraging him to take his time, get educated on his disease and its treatment options, assemble a great medical team, and choose a course of action that makes best sense to him.

Yes, cancer is a fact of life. It is a life-threatening condition that requires a lifelong commitment to keeping it at bay. A newly diagnosed man is just beginning his journey. Engage with him correctly, and he will appreciate knowing that you are here to walk beside him.

TALK WITH YOUR DOCTOR AND OTHERS

Once your cancer and its aggressiveness are identified, the subject of treatment will come up. How do you proceed? What is the best option for you?

This can be a difficult and stressful decision for many. It is also when the CaPLESS Method (CM)can be a valuable asset. No matter the course of action you choose—even if it involves not doing anything at all—the CM can provide the foundation you need for ultimate wellness and prostate cancer management.

Again, this book is not about making suggestions on what treatment approach you should take. Every case is different. But I will say this: Once you receive your diagnosis and have a complete picture of what you're up against, do not rush into a treatment. Take your time. Look at all your options. Time really is on your side. Chances are your prostate cancer will likely not spread any time soon. And this is likely the biggest decision of your life, so make sure it's the right one for you.

Here are some tips I recommend when exploring treatment:

- Consider bringing your wife or partner with you to all doctor visits. Spouses seem to have an innate ability to take good notes and ask good questions. At least this has been my clinical observation.
- Consult with at least three reputable doctors.
- Ask friends about the doctors they chose and why. You may have at least one friend who's already gone through the prostate cancer gauntlet.
- If you have no friends who have gone through prostate cancer treatment, then try visiting a prostate cancer support group. However, be cautious with any advice. If the group is one where everyone chose to have surgery, they may strongly suggest that route whether or not it is the right treatment for you. Active surveillance may be an option for you.
- Make sure at least one of the doctors you visit is associated with a reputable academic institution like NYU Langone Medical

Center, the Mayo Clinic or John's Hopkins for example. See *US News and Worlds Report's* list for the top 100 urology clinics in the United States

- Know that doctors have biases. Surgeons want to operate. Radiation oncologists want to use radiation to eradicate cancer cells. And so on. These are not for malicious or self-centered reasons, but it only reinforces the need to get several opinions.
- Also, be wary about consulting with your family and friends about your decision. It may be counterproductive because your loved ones may be too emotional in their advice. They may not understand the significance of your type and stage of prostate cancer. All they hear is cancer.

TREATMENT OPTIONS

As you explore possible treatments, you will probably hear a lot about the three most common ones: active surveillance, surgery, and radiation. Each have their upsides and downsides, but chances are one of them may be the best road for you and your prostate cancer. Remember, what works for one person may not be right for another, so you have to keep in mind several factors, such as your PSA and Gleason scores, family history, lifestyle, and psychological reaction—which one will you be most comfortable with? To help you get a head start on your treatment research, here is a summary of the top three options and what each offers:

ACTIVE SURVEILLANCE

For many men, the best treatment may be no treatment at all because more prostate cancers are discovered at an extremely early stage, thanks to widespread prostate screening. It is not a wait-and-see approach where something is done only when the cancer has advanced. In active surveillance, you won't be given any treatment unless your doctor detects early signs that the cancer is growing or becoming more aggressive. But you will have to return to the doctor regularly for blood tests, digital rectal exams and, possibly, biopsies to keep close tabs on disease progression. You also will have to pay close attention to any symptoms.

The term active surveillance is often used interchangeably with watchful waiting, but there's a big difference. Although both involve forgoing immediate therapy, watchful waiting is generally more passive, with treatment given when symptoms of cancer progression occur, whereas active surveillance patients are recommended for active therapy only when PSA and biopsy results indicate disease progression.

Active surveillance is primarily an option for those who have a cancer that is not likely to progress—such as cancer confined to the prostate—and have a low Gleason score, PSA level, and clinical stage. However, some evidence suggests that it also might be suitable for certain men with intermediate-risk prostate cancer.

The biggest drawback to active surveillance is psychological—the ongoing stress and even panic that you have cancer and are not doing anything about it. Many men cannot handle the passive approach of taking no action and have a tough time following this option. The CM can help with this problem since you're being proactive as you take action to change your eating habits, improve fitness and lifestyle, and create a inhospitable body for cancer. Even if you are not currently undergoing traditional medical treatments, you are still treating yourself.

SURGERY

Surgery to completely remove the prostate (also known as prostatectomy) is the most common treatment for prostate cancer. Today, most of these procedures are done in a way that attempts to spare the nerve bundle that control erections.

The two most common forms of surgery are retropubic radical prostatectomy (RRP) in which doctors remove the prostate through a 5–8 cm incision from your pubic bone and umbilicus (belly button) and robotic prostate removal which has gained ground in the last 10 years and is the most popular prostate surgical removal procedure.

Surgery is a simple concept for men to embrace—just take it out—which is why it's often a popular choice. In the male mind, the action plan is clear—find problem, remove problem, then be cured. Of course, it's not that simple, and surgery is big decision and can affect many aspects of you and your partner's life. Many men may not want to deal with the stress and anxiety of surgery, and there is still the chance you could face issues like incontinence and sexual problems. Even if you pick this treatment, you will need the CM protocol as your body needs help to heal, recover, and thrive so you can resume your everyday—and no doubt better—life.

RADIATION

Although radiation is generally believed to be about as effective as surgery to prevent cancer from spreading over a 10-year period, it is still unclear which treatment works better. The American Urological Association's guidelines reflect this lack of evidence, stating that both surgery and radiation are acceptable options. There are two forms of radiation, each of which carries different potential risks:

- **External-beam radiation**: the standard treatment, called external-beam radiation, uses powerful X-rays to attack the cancer. Research indicates that men who receive high-dose external beam radiation are less likely to have their cancer recur than men who get a conventional dose. However, further investigation is needed to determine whether high-dose radiation will actually save more lives than conventional-dose radiation. External-beam radiation treatments take only about 15 minutes each day, but they can still be time-consuming, as you will have to go to the treatment facility five days per week for about two months.
- **Brachytherapy**: the other form of radiation therapy is radioactive seed implants. This treatment, known as brachytherapy, works best for small- to medium-sized cancers and may reduce

the rectal symptoms of external-beam radiation. In this treatment, doctors implant small radioactive pellets into your prostate that can deliver a higher dose of radiation than external-beam radiation. Using an ultrasound-or MRI-guided needle, doctors will place an average of 100 pellets, depending on the size and shape of the prostate. The outpatient procedure takes about an hour to complete.

In the most common procedure, the pellets, which are about the size of grains of rice, remain inside you forever (although some doctors use higher-dose pellets that are left inside the prostate only temporarily). The radiation these pellets emit travels only a few millimeters, so that it is unlikely to travel beyond your prostate, thus hopefully reducing complications.

However, because the radiation is inside the prostate and closer to the urethra, brachytherapy causes urinary problems in nearly all men, and these urinary symptoms tend to be more severe than in external-beam radiation.

Some patients need a catheter to help them urinate during treatment. Evidence suggests, though, that the more active you are shortly after the brachytherapy procedure, the fewer urinary side effects you will have. (Again, another advantage to the CM as it helps to get you moving and active on a regular basis.) The radiation in the pellets can take up to a year to be completely exhausted, depending on the material used.

Radiation takes time to complete and can be an uncomfortable journey. It probably falls between active surveillance (watch and wait) and surgery (physically stressful with long and unpredictable recovery). If you do opt for radiation, you may need the CM more than ever. It can help your body cope with the procedures and improve your strength and wellness as the treatments begin to take effect and as you focus on monitoring to ensure the cancer does not return.

FOCAL RADIATION THERAPY (CYBERKNIFE)

Cyberknife: cyberknife has nothing to do with a knife, or cutting, as the name implies. It is a treatment to deliver radiotherapy with the intention of targeting treatment more accurately than standard radiotherapy. Cyberknife delivers high dose hypofractionated stereotactic body radiation therapy using a robotic arm in combination with intrafractional prostate motion tracking. A slight initial PSA increase (also called a PSA bounce) after Cyberknife is normal and is not indicative of disease progression. (Vu et al. 2015). Cyberknife is a promising technique and I expect future research will continue to support its value in the treatment of prostate cancer.

MINIMALLY INVASIVE ABLATIVE THERAPY (MIAT)

MIAT is an emerging and popular alternative group treatment option for active surveillance of patients with low-grade prostate cancer. MIAT options include: focal laser ablation, high intensive frequency ultrasound, and cryotherapy.

Here's a brief description of each, but don't make a decision on your treatment based on these summaries. This information is simply an introduction. For physicians reading this book, the department of urology at New York University holds an excellent conference every June, which provides the latest on prostate imaging and MIAT.

- **Focal Laser Ablation (FLA)** is the destruction of tissue using a focused beam of electromagnetic radiation emitted from a laser directly to the cancerous tissue with minimal destruction of normal tissue. FLA applies real-time, three-dimensional (3D) MRI technology in the focus treatment of prostate cancer. FLA poses up to a 65 percent curative rate in a small patient population with little to no urinary incontinence and sexual problems. Some of the unwanted effects include blood in the urine and semen, mild pain in the pelvic area, infection, and fever. (Lepor et al. 2015) FLA research is still maturing, but it might be an option for some types of prostate cancers.

- **High Intensity Frequency Ultrasound (HIFU)** is a where the patient is anesthetized from the waist down. A urologist controls the probe for insertion into the rectum and the device delivers ultrasound energy (similar type of energy used to see the image of a fetus during pregnancy) to a focused cancerous portion of the prostate while preserving other surrounding tissues. Low occurrences of erectile dysfunction and urinary incontinence have been reported. The main unwanted side effect is urethral stricture—the narrowing of the tube that lets out urine and semen. HIFU is an approved treatment for prostate cancer in most countries, but not yet in the United States. (Alkhorayef et al. 2015)
- **Focal Cryotherapy** works by freezing an area or the whole prostate using argon-based probes at a temperature of minus 40 degrees Celsius at the central part of the prostate and the surrounding area. Rates of urinary incontinence and impotence are low in focal cryotherapy compared to whole gland cryotherapy, where impotence rates are much higher. (Mendez et al. 2015)

MAKING THE DECISION

After you have thoroughly analyzed all your options, and listened to multiple experts, shut your brain off and spend some quiet time in reflection for about a week and see what your gut tells you. Often, a newly diagnosed patient will go through "analysis paralysis" where thought processes freeze and he chooses treatments that he later regrets. You want to avoid this kind of knee jerk decision-making.

Once you commit to a treatment and a doctor with whom you want to work, be 100 percent committed. Just as with the CM, total commitment is the only means to long-term success. Now that you have a clearer understanding of your prostate cancer and future options for treatment, let's explore in detail the inner workings of the CM and how it can help transform your life while managing your prostate cancer.

CM Profile: Larry and Claire

How CM Helped: The CaPLESS Method improved the health and well-being of both partners.

Larry is one of those men who always felt the shadow of prostate cancer. His father died from the disease, and he has diligently monitored his prostate health and made sure to act if the hint of cancer ever arose.

He had his PSA checked on a regular basis, and watched it gradually rise over the years. A biopsy confirmed a low-grade cancer, but since he caught it early, he had many options for treatment. He elected to have surgery, but realized this was not the end, only the beginning. "I wanted to be proactive about my condition and my health and knew I had to change my ways," he says.

Larry's wife, Claire, was a breast cancer survivor, so they both were engaged in learning more about cancer and post-treatment strategies. They attended a CaPLESS weekend retreat in New York to get more educated and to become more involved as a team.

"Having gone through Claire's cancer made me realize that cancer involves everyone in your life and not just you," says Larry.

What he quickly learned was that although it is easy feel alone, there are many men out there who have the same anxiety and uncertainty, and are looking for answers.

"I realized that my prostate cancer is not the same as my father's," says Larry. "It used to be hush-hush and you didn't talk about it. But now prostate cancer is out there and commonly accepted, and when you can have that open conversation you no longer see cancer as scary, but as something you can do something about."

Adds Claire: "It was eye-opening to see other people talk about how they changed their lifestyle with better nutrition and fitness and that they were survivors. It is so good for men, and the women, to see and hear that, and to realize that there is a way not only to live, but have a better life."

Another takeaway for Larry was that the CM taught him that you do not need to make huge changes to experience big changes in your life. He realized that doing something every day, even if it seems small, adds up. "I do a minimal amount of exercise each day–50 push-ups, sit-ups, and cycling. It is a regimen, like brushing your teeth–so it does not feel like work, but just part of daily life."

CHAPTER 2

WELCOME TO THE CAPLESS METHOD

I would rather know the person who has the disease than the disease a person has.

—*Hippocrates*

In 2002, colon cancer struck down one of the country's leading urologists, William Fair M.D. Dr. Fair was a well-respected prostate cancer surgeon and chairman of urology at Memorial Sloan-Kettering Cancer Center (MSKCC) in New York, from 1984 until 1997. He was first diagnosed in 1995 and began treatment at MSKCC, which is regarded as one of the country's top cancer institutions for surgery and chemotherapy.

He was in the best hands possible. He went under the knife to remove some of his cancerous colon and was fine for a while, but in 1997 the cancer returned, and he endured a second surgery. Soon his cancer was labeled "aggressive and incurable" and his doctor gave him a 1 in 10 chance to live five years.

"My choices were limited—another risky operation, extensive radiation, and experimental chemotherapy," Fair told *The New York Times*. "Knowing these treatments could be very toxic and debilitating, I set out on my own to investigate approaches outside conventional medicine that I felt would preserve my quality of life, and perhaps slow the progression of the disease."

Dr. Fair, a respected scientist and surgeon who once called complementary medicine, "touchy-feely West Coast nonsense," decided to take a more natural approach to his treatment. He made major dietary changes, adopted a regular yoga practice and exercise routine, and embraced various herbal supplements.

This new approach to his life worked. It did not cure his cancer, but Fair was able to remain active until a few weeks before his death—five years after he was given a mere 10 percent chance of living five years.

Even his doctor, Murray F. Brennan, M.D., was shocked by his longevity. "I think everyone was surprised at how long he lived," he said later. "Certainly whatever he was doing didn't do any harm either."

I often wonder what would have happened if Dr. Fair began his complementary treatments when he was first diagnosed. Would he have lived a longer and healthier life? Would his cancer have regressed? Would he still be around today? Hard to tell, but I speculate his outcome would have been even better with earlier lifestyle interventions.

Why is Fair's story so important? I believe we can learn three fundamental points from his experience:

1. He lived much longer than anyone anticipated with an aggressive cancer.
2. He apparently had good quality of life until the very end.
3. The intelligent combination of natural medicine with conventional medicine (that is, integrative medicine) works well.

Of course, everyone is different. No two people will experience the same results, but Fair's story illustrates the power of an open mind and the power of lifestyle medicine. Fair bypassed the traditional Western medicine he practiced for decades, and embraced a treatment program that was easy to implement, and showed positive results. And as his physician pointed out, it did not harm him in any way or cause any negative side effects. His quality of life improved and he was able to stave off succumbing to his cancer longer than anyone thought possible.

Lifestyle Modification to Reduce Prostate Cancer Progression—the Ornish Trials

Dr. Dean Ornish is arguably the most renowned researcher on lifestyle and nutritional interventions against prostate cancer.

His approach follows four components: A diet high in whole foods, plant-- based protein, fruits, vegetables, unrefined grains, and legumes, and low in fat (approximately 10 percent of calories) and refined carbohydrates; moderate aerobic exercise (walking 30 minutes per day, six days per week); stress management (gentle yoga--based stretching, breathing, meditation, imagery, and progressive relaxation for 60 minutes daily); increased social support (60 minutes of weekly support--group sessions).

A large part of the CaPLESS Method is borrowed from Dr. Ornish's research on lifestyle and prostate cancer. And research has shown this approach to be quite effective. Here is a look at some of Dr. Ornish's latest research.

In one study, Dr. Ornish and his team examined 93 men with early biopsy-proven prostate cancer who volunteered to skip radiation, chemotherapy, and surgery for their disease. Instead, he separated them into two groups. One group (the treatment group) followed a lifestyle modification protocol.The other group served as a control group, and did not make any diet or lifestyle changes..

By the end of the yearlong study, six of the control group (the non-lifestyle group) had dropped out because their tumors were growing. However, not one of the lifestyle group participants suffered the same fate. After two years of follow--up, 13 of the 49 non-lifestyle participants (27 percent) had undergone conventional prostate cancer treatment (radical prostatectomy, radiation therapy, or androgen deprivation). In comparison only two of the 43 members of the lifestyle group underwent some kind of treatment. (Ornish et al. 2005)

Another nonrandomized trial run by Dr. Ornish and his team, called the Gene Expression Modulation by Intervention with Nutrition and Lifestyle (GEMINAL) study, looked at 30 men with indolent low-risk prostate cancers. The researchers found a significant improvement in cardiovascular disease risk, including reductions in weight loss, blood pressure, and cholesterol levels. Waist size also shrank by about three inches, and triglycerides and C-reactive protein—an inflammatory marker—also slightly decreased.

Lastly, Dr. Ornish looked at the men with low-risk prostate cancer and their telomere length after five years. Telomeres help protect DNA, and studies show keeping telomeres long protects cells from aging, cancer, and premature death.

Shortened telomeres have been linked with an increased risk of prostate cancer recurrence after surgery. Dr. Ornish found that his lifestyle intervention was associated with increases in relative telomere length after a five-year follow up. (Ornish et al. 2013)

THE CAPLESS METHOD –WHAT IS IT?

I believe Dr. Fair was on to something, especially at a time (circa 1995) when natural medicine wasn't as popular as it is now. He showed that there was a different approach to cancer treatment and co-management. It does not just have to be about radiation and surgery.

You see, mainstream medicine does not build health—although it's part of the *healthcare* system. Worthy as it may be, it only attempts to treat disease. It's a fight of us versus them. A war. Find cancer, kill cancer.

Yes, those approaches are at times necessary, but they do not always have to be the first move—much less the only the move. At some point someone or something needs to treat you, the patient—the host of the cancer. You need to become physically and biochemically stronger so that your biological soil is hostile to cancer.

Dr. Fair tackled his cancer from the perspective that one's lifestyle choices may be the best medicine. As a longtime naturopathic doctor who follows the guidelines of natural medicine, I knew this was not a new concept by any means, but I wanted to further explore the link between Fair's actions and his results—especially since he was a renowned prostate cancer physician and surgeon. Would it work for other kinds of cancer, especially my area of interest: prostate cancer?

I spent over a decade researching how diet, exercise, and supplementation affected cancer. I dug through hundreds of scientific journals, and examined books on virtually every type of cancer from the Budwig diet to macrobiotic and everything in between. I looked at what worked, what didn't, and most importantly, why. After years of refining and tweaking—adding more of this, less of that, and closely observing how my patients responded—I developed an all-around natural, easy-to-follow lifestyle approach to prostate cancer: the CaPLESS Method (CM). It is based on five pillars I found to be most successful in treating and managing prostate cancer: eating, exercise (movement), supplementation, stress management, and sleep.

Now, you don't have to be perfect at all of these at that same time, but you do want to work toward perfection. In other words, some days you will fall off the dietary horse, but get good movement in, and do well in lowering stress and getting plenty of sleep. Other times you'll remember to take your supplements and eat well, but forget to exercise for a day or more. That's OK. The goal is to assess and improve. The CM is not an all-or-nothing program.

Now, I did not invent the various aspects of this program. Each element has existed before, and has a strong scientific support of success. I simply examined the evidence related to lifestyle modification and prostate cancer and took the components that worked best—from diet to exercise to supplementation—and put it all together as a practical guide for men with prostate cancer to follow.

Your partner and family can apply these methods, too. In fact, they will also enjoy mental clarity, abundance of energy, and good lab reports from their physician.

When it comes to medical treatment, we still cling to the mindset that there is only one approach: cut it out or zap it with radiation. Instead, the CM is designed to focus on multiple pathways of treating and managing prostate cancer with the idea that an arsenal approach is stronger than a single one. In other words, we throw the kitchen sink at prostate cancer so your body naturally discourages healthy cells from going wild uncontrollably like cancer cells.

The ultimate goal of the CM is to create a microenvironment hostile to cancer cells. Think of it as creating biological soils in your body so weeds (cancer) do not grow, and those already there may even shrivel and die.

But the CM is not only about managing your prostate cancer. It's a game plan to help you embrace a robust lifestyle and prevent dying early from anything else. Your prostate cancer diagnosis becomes an opportunity to thrive, not just survive. By following the program you reap many other benefits along the way: healthy weight loss, jolts of energy, and improved heart health—all areas that can lead to other health problems as you age if not monitored, and that can affect you long before prostate cancer does. Specifically, at a cellular, DNA level, the CM can do the following to promote greater health and wellness:

- reduce oxidative stress
- lower chronic inflammation

- improve detoxification capacity
- strengthen the immune system
- control sugar levels and insulin production

By controlling these five cellular elements, you will reduce your chances of forming more dangerous cancer cells, reduce your chances of dying prematurely, and live your best life moving forward.

WHAT'S IN A NAME?

So many diets and wellness programs focus on the don't—don't eat this, don't do that, don't take this. This approach to eating is simply unsustainable and why diets don't work. People feel deprived and not fulfilled. In comparison, the CaPLESS Method focuses on the dos—do eat more of this, do more of that, and do less of the other.

Also, I provide the Lowest Effective Dose (LED) and Maximal Safe Amount (MSA) of the individual pillars. What is that? Wouldn't you want to know the minimal amount of foods, movement, supplements, sleep, etc., you need to get maximal results? I do, which is why I offer the LED I also want to know what is the highest, safe amount of chocolate cake I can have—the MSA.

So exactly what is the CaPLESS Method? Here is how the acronym breaks down:

"CaP"—carcinoma of the prostate: Once again, this is the medical term for prostate cancer.

"L"—lifestyle: This refers to how you live. By modifying your behavior you become more aware of your habits and can begin to make healthier daily choices.

"E" —eating and exercise/movement:

The focus here is not only on what food not to eat, but what food to eat. I examined all the popular and effective diets from Dean Ornish's full spectrum to Johanna Budwig's diet to macrobiotic to Paleo. Then I extracted what I believe are the best parts and folded them into a new eating plan that focuses on the right foods and ingredients that will create a hostile environment for cancer cells, as well as protect your body from other potentially debilitating health problems.

Movement and exercise is equally important. We are simply not made to sit for long periods. We are built to move. Humans need to exercise, plain and simple. It does not matter what exercise you choose as long as you do something. However, the key is to get out of your comfort zone and challenge yourself. You need to build up a good sweat at all times. You need to mix it up and try different routines that work different muscles. And even after you work out, you still need to stay active. Studies show that if you exercise 60 minutes a day, but are sedentary the rest of the time, you are still not reaching your protective potential. Exercise is not something you do for a fixed time and then forget about it. You need to make a conscious effort to sit less and stay active throughout the day. I know work can be interference, but the CM can make it realistic and sustainable for you.

"S"—supplementation: I have long been a proponent of the right mix of dietary supplements for the right person at the right time. I believe in them so much that I take more than 20 every day for additional protection. I am convinced they have a necessary role in improving health and creating a hostile cancer environment. When it comes to men with prostate cancer, the right supplement combination is essential.

But you have to be smart about your supplementation. I often see patients take too many dietary supplements that have more downside than upside. Some are actually promoting cancer. Not all supplements are right for you and not just any kind of supplement will be appropriate.

Nowadays, you can take multivitamins that contain almost every kind of vitamin and mineral (and the generic versions are really cheap, too). But is that what you need? Or you hear a news story that says a particular vitamin is harmful, so you immediately stop taking it without any idea if that is the right move for you, or even if the study the story was based on is accurate. What dietary supplements to take and not to take can be confusing. But keep in mind that while the right supplement regimen is an integral part of the CM arsenal, it's not designed to be a substitute for proper nutrition.

"S"—sleep and stress: It seems like not a day goes by that I do not read about another study voicing the importance of sleep to one's health. We don't get enough, plain and simple. We have this crazy idea that we can get by with less sleep. Some men even brag about the fact they only need five hours of sleep per night. It's like a badge of honor for them. That way of thinking is foolish. When you are constantly going without restorative sleep, your body does not work as well.

When it's tired, it cannot do its jobs as effectively. When it comes to prostate cancer, you need your body to be rested and ready to fight at all times. And when you are well rested, you are able to better manage stress.

The word "stress" gets casually tossed around. "My job stresses me out!" Stress is real, and research has shown that when we are under constant stress, the body produces too much cortisol—the stress hormone—that triggers ongoing inflammation and makes it more difficult for the body to fight invaders like prostate cancer. Sleep and stress go hand-in-hand. You need to embrace healthier sleep patterns and adopt stress-reducing techniques. They are both essential for optimal wellness. And I know some readers may suffer from long-term insomnia. I get it. For thousands of people worldwide, it's not easy to sleep well. With some tools and techniques, I hope to show you how.

THE CAPLESS METHOD IN ACTION

How do I know the CM works? Because I have seen the results with thousands of patients and CaPLESS retreat attendees. For the past several years,

I have hosted weekend CaPLESS Wellness retreats in and around New York City for men diagnosed with prostate cancer and their life partners. Over a two-day period, men and their significant others give up their weekends to immerse themselves in learning and applying the CM into their lives.

A natural gourmet chef shows how to select ingredients and prepare meals based on the CaPLESS eating philosophy (as well as how not to fear the kitchen). Participants are taught principles of yoga and how to breathe and use their bodies to best manage stress. Our exercise physiologist instructs attendees on how to begin and maintain a vigorous exercise routine based on individual cancer diagnosis and fitness level. And perhaps best of all, the men are given hands-on guidance on how to begin to make lasting change.

Between patients at the clinic and our retreat attendees I have witnessed the power of this anti-cancer lifestyle approach countless times. I've seen firsthand how a well-executed lifestyle plan generates a mental shift from a life of only surviving to one of thriving. I know it's a challenge to reverse years of behavior and habits that interfere with you staying cancer-free and you cannot do that over a single weekend, but you can take the first steps in the right direction.

After these retreats, I do follow up visits with the men to assess their status, discuss challenges, and tailor the program to better fit their individual lifestyles. I have witnessed many remarkable changes since they began following the CaPLESS program. Some have rediscovered their lost energy and mental outlook. Some have melted excess cancer-causing fat from their bodies for the first time in ages. And perhaps best of all, some have even found that their prostate cancer has stalled—and in some cases even reversed.

You will read many of their stories in this book, and hopefully, you will relate to many of them. They are men just like you who face the same challenges and confront the same fears. By hearing from men just like yourself, you can begin to see how this program can help you manage your prostate cancer, and how the CM can help you not only survive, but thrive.

CAPLESS METHOD AND PROSTATE CANCER—WHAT IS THE CONNECTION?

Now you may think, "This all sounds good, but how can it help me cure my prostate cancer or even prevent a recurrence after medical treatment?" Good question. Just because something is supposed to work, does not mean it will, right?

To understand the connection between the CM and your prostate cancer you have to understand first *why* you have cancer. When you can understand how prostate cancer develops then can you see the how the CM helps.

So how can you go most of your life with no health problems and then one day out of the blue—BAM!—you are told you have prostate cancer?

First off, cancer is a disease where cells grow and divide uncontrollably. If these aberrant cells stay local and do not move, then you either cut it out or zap it with some form of energy like radiation to prevent it from moving to other organs. If the cancer cells are low level, as in a Gleason 6 prostate cancer, then active surveillance may be an option. If cancer cells move outside of the prostate, these cells invade and destroy other tissues like the bones or lungs. What makes the cells behave like this? Although the answer can be complicated, the interplay between your environment and your genetics seem to be one of the main culprits.

Genes are found in every single cell in your body, and there are about 30,000 in each cell. They determine everything from the color of your hair and eyes to your height and even how long you may live. You cannot change your genes. They come from your parents. In essence, you were dealt your life's hand the day you were born.

Unfortunately, genes often indicate whether you may eventually get cancer or some other kind of disease. For instance, if you have the diabetes gene from your parents, then you are more likely to develop diabetes. If you have the prostate cancer gene from your father, you are more likely to get prostate cancer.

So is there nothing you can do? Are you doomed for being born to the wrong parents? While you cannot change your genes—or your parents—it may be possible to change how your genes behave.

THE INSIDE STORY OF GENES

Let's take a closer look at genes and how they work. Genes are made of deoxyribonucleic acid, or as you may know it: DNA. Genes control how a cell functions, including how quickly it grows, how often it divides, and how long it lives. To control these functions, genes produce proteins that perform specific tasks and act as messengers for the cell. Therefore, it is essential that each gene have the correct instructions, or code, for making its protein so the protein can do the right job.

It is like following a recipe. You need the right ingredients in the right amount to make the right meal. But if that recipe gets altered—i.e., your DNA changes—that can set off a reaction in your genes that causes your cells to go haywire. Cancer can develop, and if not stopped, can grow and spread until it eventually overwhelms your body.

So in order to stop and control your prostate cancer, you have to create a new meal.

EPIGENETICS AND PROSTATE CANCER

This is where epigenetics come in. I know it sounds like something from your high school science book, but epigenetics are key to your prostate cancer. Epigenetics allow you to control which gene you express at any one time. And prostate cancer management is all about modifying a gene's DNA recipe. By adding or eliminating certain nutrients to or from your body's genes, you can shake up your DNA and manipulate how your cells behave. This means you can control whether or not cancer or other diseases develop, or if disease does develop, you may be able to slow, stop, or perhaps even reverse its progression. Put simply—you are not destined to encounter prostate cancer, or any other disease, based on your genes alone. Instead, you can create your own health destiny based on the science of epigenetics.

Within the last 20 years, the evolving science of epigenetics has shown that several factors and processes—specifically environmental chemicals, lifestyle choices, and diet—affect your genes. By changing your exposure to these items you can manipulate your DNA, create a new recipe, and like a light switch, dim the genes that cause prostate cancer. Epigenetics do not change your DNA, but they can alter how DNA behaves within your genes.

This is where the CaPLESS Method comes into play. By adopting its five pillar principles, you can keep out the bad stuff that affects your DNA and invite in the good stuff to help make a new and healthier DNA recipe. It is much like a New York City apartment building doorman who determines who comes in and who stays out.

NOTE TO LIFE PARTNER

This is one of the most important parts of your man's overall journey with prostate cancer. At this point in his diagnosis, he will feel overwhelmed with this new direction in his life. Everything is foreign as he begins to make significant changes in his life. New eating plan? Exercise regimen? Supplements? Although the CM strives to reduce stress, beginning this program can induce some temporary stress. That's part of the process. But he will be more successful at embracing this new lifestyle if you join him. Tell him you will also adopt the CM. And believe me, you will benefit from it, too. If you are on board, he won't feel alone. No need to feel pressured. Just enjoy the journey and remember to be patient with him. You don't want to take the lead and be pushy–don't knock a cookie out of his hand, or ask him every day if he worked out. Let him determine his speed and progress. Some men take longer to implement change than others. Just be there for him. Give him wiggle room. Guide him intelligently. He needs to be in charge and always feel he's making the decisions to eat better and work out. The more he does, the more comfortable he will become, and the more successful he will be. Remember: You are not making the decisions for him.

HOW THE CAPLESS METHOD WORKS

In the following chapters, you will learn in detail how each of the five pillars of the CM work: eating, movement, supplementation, and stress and sleep management. You will see how they each relate to prostate cancer, what the science says and how they support each other to create that strong foundation and make that hostile microenvironment to combat your prostate cancer. These elements also work to renew your energy, lose extra pounds, think clearer, be fitter, and live a more vibrant life.

Remember, prostate cancer is not the end, but the beginning of a new way to live and thrive.

After you have learned about the CM's five pillars then it is time to put it into action. It begins with a 21 Day Reset, which helps jump-start your body so you can flush out those built-up toxins, begin to sweat and exercise, clear your mind, and feed your body the vital foods and nutrients it now needs. This is the CM in action and will help you learn how to implement into your daily life so it becomes a habit and part of who you are and how you live.

TO-GO MESSAGE

Your prostate cancer can be a blessing in disguise. It is a wake-up call that you need to make significant changes—not just to manage your cancer, but to improve your quality of life. See your diagnosis as an opportunity to revamp how you eat, how you exercise, and even how you think.

Prostate cancer is not the end—it is the beginning.

This is your chance to take control of your life, reexamine how you have lived and adopt a new lifestyle that not only can help you accept your diagnosis and perhaps improve your condition, but can also reduce your risk of other health conditions.

This is the ultimate cause-and-effect strategy. You do this and you get that result. You do something positive and you have a positive effect. You have the power to change you behavior, your mind-set, and your health. Don't be a victim of prostate cancer. Thrive—don't only survive.

In the next chapter, I will show you the first step in the CM, revamping your eating habits, and why what you do eat is just as important as what you don't eat.

CM Profile: Chad, age 49

How CM Helped: Chad was able to change his life in order to spend more quality time with his children.

At age 46, Chad became a father again—but not in the traditional way. He and his wife already had three kids together, ages 21, 18, and 14, and they were looking to become foster parents.

"We were looking for a six-year-old, but the agency called and said they had a three-day-old baby boy who needed a home, so we said "yes," he says.

When I met Chad, he had a PSA of 28.1ng/ml. His prostate biopsy revealed: Multiple positive cores with Gleason scores: 9, 8 and 7 (4+3). Shortly after, he underwent a prostatectomy. When he returned to see me after his procedure on October 2012, his first post-surgery PSA, we were surprised, did not budge much - it was 20.2ng/ml. (this is not a typo).

After a year as foster parents, they officially adopted the baby. As part of the adoption process, Chad was required to get a physical. He took a PSA test and it came back with an astronomical score of 27. A few retests confirmed the number and he had a biopsy, which revealed full-blown cancer.

The choice was easy for him—surgery—and he had it a week after the adoption became final. "I like to think that I helped to save this baby, but in fact, he saved mine," says Chad.

He soon adopted the CM as part of his post-surgery recovery. The CM taught him to think beyond his middle-aged desk job lifestyle. "Before, I weighed 205 pounds and had a travel-heavy job that filled me up on red meat, white bread, and zero exercise."

He embraced the CM plan 100 percent and learned how easy it was to eat smarter without sacrificing what he loved. For instance, he discovered he could still enjoy the occasional chicken wings, only now he has organic meat, baked and not fried, with sugar-free barbeque sauce.

He avoided the trappings of business dinners by swap out or remove out or take out ingredients on the menu—no cheese, dressings on the side, and a salad instead of a big potato.

After following the CM for six months, his PSA numbers dropped from 20 to four. Today, it is less than 0.1. His high cholesterol and acid reflux have vanished. He rises early, goes to bed on time. "I have found that there are two roads you can take: give up or do not give up. I choose the latter and do everything I can to live a quality life as long as I can."

Along with hormone deprivation therapy, Chad is diligent about the CaPLESS approach. Today Chad is a vibrant, slim and fit 50 year-old with an undetectable PSA, running a successful business and with a load of energy.

CHAPTER 3

CAPLESS EATING: SUSTAINABLE, ENJOYABLE, AND PROTECTIVE

Eat food. Not too much. Mostly plants.

—MICHAEL POLLAN

I HAVE NEVER been a fan of the word diet. Just look at the word—right smack in the middle is DIE! No one likes to DIEt and no one sticks to one. A diet suggests a temporary, arduous program with a specific goal in mind. "I'm going on a diet for two weeks to lose 20 pounds for the wedding or reunion." You follow it, maybe hit your goal, and then toss it aside.

Diet also can mean being deprived. If you think about a diet, what comes to mind? A lot of NO!—No, you can't eat this, and no you can't eat that. It is not enjoyable. It feels unnatural, stressful, and limited. Who wants to live like that? I don't. That's a main reason many popular diets are not successful for the long haul. They are just quick fixes without lasting results.

This is why I created a specific way of eating as a lifestyle change—and not a temporary situation. I want it to become part of who you are and something you follow for the rest of your life. You have to eat every day to survive, but why make it something that is designed to be limited? It doesn't make sense. In the same way you may identify yourself by your profession—entrepreneur, attorney, truck driver—I want you to think of yourself as a CaPLESS thriver. This is a man living his best life yet despite, and in spite of his prostate cancer. And it begins with what you put in your mouth. So let's begin.

CAPLESS EATING

The connection between diet and cancer has been revealing itself for decades. The first scientific research linking the relationship between food and cancer appeared in 1981. Since then tons of follow ups have dug deeper into this concept and discovered not only what foods (and specific ingredients) can help prevent cancer, but also what may slow or even reverse its progression.

What you eat matters. Some of my patients boast about how healthy they eat so they don't understand why they got prostate cancer. Sadly, I have come to realize that no one knows what healthy eating means anymore. Virtually every one is confused about this. One day eating low fat with lots of soy is the way to go; the next day it's high protein and low carb. It is confusing and even frustrating. If you think you eat healthy for the most part, I would bet there is plenty you neglect to prevent, manage, or reduce your chances of a recurrence.

CaPLESS eating is a different way to think about food. It is about eating to live—not living to eat. It's about eating real food. It's about loving the journey to eat the cleanest and freshest foods possible and appreciate how fantastic you feel because of it—a slimmer, stronger body with plenty of energy, and a sharper mind.

This way of eating is not about following recipes, one after the other, but rather educating yourself so you can identify the good and bad foods, whether you are at the grocery store or eating out, so you can begin to make better choices. You will learn what foods can and can't help fight prostate cancer and which foods also can reduce your risk of heart disease and other illnesses.

Now to be clear, I'm not against all diets—just the opposite. I think many diet plans, such as plant-based, low glycemic, Mediterranean and paleo, have helpful components. They all advocate some aspect of either healthy food choices or behavior modification, and most are based on solid science.

I have taken the best parts of these diet plans, along with my own research on food, nutrition, and prostate cancer, and folded them into a comprehensive strategy, which I simply call CaPLESS eating. It is easy to follow, sustainable, and most important is scientifically based to help manage, slow, and perhaps even reverse your prostate cancer.

Eating should not be complicated. In fact, humans used to eat simply. Our ancestors consumed meals rich in fat and protein, and low, but not completely devoid, of unrefined carbohydrates. They included ingredients found in the dirt, on trees, and grazing in the fields—not made in a laboratory. But as society became industrialized, diets became more processed with the emphasis on faster cooking and cheaper ingredients including chemicals, artificial flavors, and additives. The continuous rise in deadly diseases is how we have paid the price.

With so much junk in our food, it is no surprise there has been a steady increase in obesity, cardiovascular disease, and yes even cancer. In fact, one recent study examined the effect of a typical ancestral diet of lean meat, vegetables, and nuts in non-obese healthy subjects versus the consumption of a typical Western diet. The researchers found significant reductions in blood pressure, plasma insulin, glucose, total cholesterol, and triglycerides among those who followed the simpler ancestral diet. I mention this prostate and cancer study because a good heart-health program is an antiprostate cancer program, too.

The bottom line is that, in order for you to take full control of your health, you have to embrace better eating. This is not something you dabble in, or only follow part time. You need to change how you approach food all together. Change how you think about food. The good news: it is not as hard as you think.

Dr. Geo's Ten Simple Rules to Eating:

1. Don't eat ANY food with guilt. Guilt is much more indigestible.

2. Don't eat until you have the full feeling. Stop before you get there.

3. If bugs would not eat it, it's probably not good for you.

4. Good food spoils. If it doesn't spoil within two weeks at room temperature, it's crap.

5. If the ingredients list is more than four unpronounceable words, it's probably crap.

6. Cut out white foods: sugar, white rice, white bread, white pasta, etc. (An exception is cauliflower, which is an awesome 5 white food.)

7. Drink clean water, good tea, and freshly squeezed juices. Some coffee is OK.

8. Learn proper portion control. It's OK to leave food on your plate—your mom will never know.

9. Eat plenty of plants with every meal.

10. If you are going to have ice cream or any other low-level food, have the real thing. The fake stuff (low-fat yogurt instead of ice cream, for example) is more damaging. If you eat it with guilt, read the first rule again.

CUT OUT THE CRAP!

CaPLESS eating is based on the basic mathematic formula of addition and subtraction. You eat much less of the bad stuff and add much more of the good stuff. It is that simple.

The bad foods, or crap as I like to call it, are often those instant gratification items usually filled with sugar and artificial ingredients. I understand why you enjoy them. They taste great and are so comforting during stressful times. Actually, they work similarly to drugs. Yep, you are actually getting high when you indulge in processed, high-sugar foods. And that indulgence comes at a hefty price.

When these toxic foods become a regular part of your diet, it can lead to chronic inflammation, weight gain, and life-threatening disease. All of these aggravate your prostate cancer as well as expose you to other illnesses, some even more dangerous than prostate cancer.

The crap is often easy to identify—you can probably list the foods you know you shouldn't eat—but there are some you may think are good for you, that aren't. For example, whole wheat bread, a simple refined carbohydrate, is a big no-no, even though it appears healthy. The real obstacle is when you don't know what to replace these foods with. Same with most fruit juices, which seem nutritious, but are just highly sugared drinks. Cutting out that double-cheeseburger value meal sounds easy, but if you don't have a suitable substitute ready, it's tough to make the change. That's why you need to both add and subtract at the same time.

I have designed a food rating system for exactly this purpose, which I will introduce in a moment. As you will see, quality additions include foods like cold-water fish, grass-fed meats, colorful fruits and vegetables, and plenty of herbs and spices. Simply add more of these, and other cancer-fighting choices, to replace what you subtract from your diet.

It is not always so simple. Some foods that might look healthy, aren't, and others may not seem beneficial, but may be the strongest weapons against your prostate cancer.

This is where the CaPLESS Food Rating System comes into play. This simple five-point rating helps you separate the good stuff from the crap by giving everything you eat a rating of 1 to 5. This way you don't have to memorize a long food list of good and bad choices. Instead, it helps to reinforce the idea of good versus bad. This way you can look at a food, or even complete meals, and immediately know if it helps or hurts your cancer management, and if you should eat it more, less, or occasionally. Here is how the CaPLESS Food Rating System breaks down:

5—Strong science support in term of anti-cancer properties. These are high-level foods you want to consume as often as possible.

4—Some science support, with ingredients that are protective against prostate cancer and other aging conditions. These are moderate-level foods you want to consume liberally.

3—Neutrals. They do not promote or protect against prostate cancer and other disease. Consume moderately and keep portions low.

2—Some science shows to directly or indirectly increase or worsen prostate cancer risk and contribute to many common diseases. You should avoid as much as possible, and when consumed, keep portions small.

1—Strong science indicates directly or indirectly increases or worsens cancer risk and contributes most to disease. You want to avoid them at all costs, if possible, or consume super moderately and in small portions.

As you can see, the higher numbers are the best and the lower ones the worst. So CaPLESS eating is about consuming more 4s and 5s, some 3s, and few 2s and 1s. This not only helps improve your eating habits, but feeds your body the nutrients it needs to create that hostile microenvironment for your cancer.

When you follow this CaPLESS 21-Day Reset as part of your introduction into the CM, you will notice that all the meals are based on this five-point system, so you can begin to make the connection between the good and the bad. After the 21-day period, you will learn to look at any food choice and know where it falls on the scale. Plate of hot wings with creamy ranch sauce: that's a 1; organic spinach salad topped with broccoli, tomatoes, and onions with olive oil, balsamic, and lemon on the side: a solid 5.

Understanding this will also help you indulge every now and then — guilt-free. As my clinical nutrition professor said in naturopathic medical school years ago, "Guilt is more indigestible than any cookie."

CaPLESS eating is not an "exclusion" diet—no-fat this, low carb that, drink only this. It's about eating real food as frequently possible. Those exclusionary diets have proven to be boring and unsustainable. Besides, it's human nature to want more of what you can't have, isn't it? My two year-old always wants my cell phone more than his favorite toy. Reaching for "the forbidden fruit" is practically a hardwired behavior

If you always say to yourself, "I can't have donuts, I can't have donuts, I can't have donuts," then donuts are what you will crave. So, yes, you can have a donut—once in a while. You just need to make sure it's a sometime food, not an everyday food like Cookie Monster once said. (Yes, I still watch *Sesame Street* with my kids.) And when you do enjoy the occasional junk food, you will know to place a rating of 1 next to it and realize that your next meal should contain a lot of 4s and 5s to balance it out.

A Note To Your Life Partner

This part of the CaPLESS Eating Program may be the most challenging. CaPLESS eating is not a diet. It is a lifestyle. It is different than anything he may have tried in the past whether it is the Atkins or Paleo diet. He may have some resistance to change. All men do, especially as we get older. The good news is that since CaPLESS eating is not a diet in the classic sense, it is all-inclusive, meaning you can benefit from it, too. What can help with his cancer also can help lower your risk of diseases like breast cancer. So make CaPLESS eating a group effort, a family function. Shop together, cook together, and explore new meals and recipes together. The kitchen can be a therapeutic place for both of you and for your relationship. If he sees that you are onboard and it is a true team effort, he will be much more receptive to embracing this new way of eating. Eating less and fasting 12 hours per day will likely be tough for him—especially if he finds comfort in eating late at night. Once or twice a week, he can break the rules: fast for 9 or 10 hours a night, even pig out if he wants to. In other words, once you and he know the rules and principles of this program, you can break them intelligently. But don't be too militant and tell him what to eat or to stop eating after eight o'clock all the time. Men don't like to be told what to do. Just make it a lifestyle where intelligent methods of breaking the rules are allowed. And if he wants to eat a 1 or 2 food, let him and don't judge him. If he is eating 1s and 2s excessively, gently lead him the right way, but don't hit his hand when he picks up a donut—that may not go well.

SIX BASIC PRINCIPLES OF CAPLESS EATING

So where do the 5 and 4 foods and meals come from? CaPLESS eating is also based on six key food principles and are at the foundation of all CaPLESS meal plans. You may already be familiar with many of these while others may be entirely new concepts. Yet, they comprise a vast majority of the types of 4s and 5s you need to consume on a regular basis.

This philosophy is not pulled from thin air, but based on my personal research, clinical experience, and the latest science from peer-reviewed journals. All of them are essential to create a microenvironment hostile to cancer and build the type of eating lifestyle you need to combat age-related diseases. Here is a look at each of the six and why they are so important.

1. plant foods
2. organic
3. eat less
4. good fish
5. raw nuts and seeds
6. herbs and spices

PLANT FOODS

What to Do: Eat more plant foods with bright colors. Stay away from white foods, like pasta, bread, and rice.

Why You Need It: The different colors of fruits and vegetables on your plate represent key plant chemicals called phytochemicals that offer protection against cancer and heart disease. Phytochemicals are what makes strawberries red, spinach green, blueberries blue, and carrots and sweet potatoes orange. These phytochemicals, specifically carotenoids like beta-carotene and lycopene, seem to offer more protection than any other agents in food. Cruciferous vegetables are particularly protective against prostate cancer and include: cabbage, broccoli, cauliflower, Brussels sprouts, Bok choy, kale, arugula, and collard greens. They are rich in nutrients called glucosinolates, sulforaphane, and indole-3 carbinol (I3C).

They increase the production of antioxidant enzymes that can protect cells from oxidative damage. (Garikapaty et al. 2005)

One recent study, which involved 600 men, found that eating three or more servings of cruciferous vegetables per week reduced their risk of newly diagnosed prostate cancer by 41 percent compared with those who consumed less than one serving per week. (Cohen et al. 2000) Another study in the *International Journal of Cancer* (Aug 5, 2011) examined 1,560 men with prostate cancer, and found that those with a high intake of cruciferous vegetables reduced their risk of their cancer growing and spreading. (Richman et al. 2011) Upping your cruciferous veggies also can lower your cardiovascular disease mortality by 31 percent, according to another study. (Zhang et al 2011)

Eat It: Focus on mixing in different colors with every meal. Think of it this way: More colors equal less cancer.

When not to Eat it: CaPLESS thrivers who develop kidney stones should consider staying away from vegetables that are only high in oxalates. These include spinach, rhubarb, beets, and Swiss chard. Other high oxalate vegetables should be consumed since the benefits outweigh the risk.

ORGANIC

What to do: Eat organic fruits and vegetables as often as possible. Yes, eating *any* fruits and vegetables is better than eating none. But certain fruits and vegetables are particularly high in pesticides and herbicides, which are also potential carcinogens (Smith-Spangler et al. 2012)

Why you need it: Pesticides and herbicides, like methyl bromide and organophosphates, have been linked to prostate cancer. While the evidence has made associations rather than a direct cause and effect link between prostate cancer and the chemicals sprayed on veggies and fruits, there is sufficient confirmation for anyone with prostate cancer to be cautious.

Eat it: The Environmental Working Group (EWG) has published and updated their Dirty Dozen Plus list showing the most chemically sprayed fruits and vegetables that should thus be eaten organically. Foods that should **always** be organic include spinach, apples, and strawberries. Foods that are OK to eat nonorganically include cauliflower, broccoli, and avocados. Read the full list at www.ewg.org.

When not to eat it: Organic fruits and vegetables can cost an average of $1 to $2 a day per person. This can be up to an additional $650 a year for one person, a significant amount for many families. If the additional price is a concern, then try to eat the fruits and vegetables on the EWG "clean fifteen" list of foods that are not high in pesticides.

EAT LESS

What to do: Don't eat for a 12-hour period from night to morning. For instance, 8:00 p.m. to 8:00 a.m. or 7:00 p.m. to 7:00 a.m., whichever works best for you.

Why you need it: Eating less has been shown to lower inflammation, reduce levels of cancer forming chemical like Insulin Like Growth Factor 1 (IGF-1) and help with weight loss. Fasting two to three hours before bedtime also improves quality of sleep.

Eat it: Eat for 12 hours a day, two or three meals a day, mostly foods ranked 3, 4, or 5. Then fast for 12 hours, including when you sleep. If weight loss is not a major issue for you—for instance, you are naturally lean—then eat high-calorie 3, 4, and 5 foods as often as possible, including nuts and nut butters, avocado, and quality meats.

When not to Eat less: Those rapidly losing weight with advanced prostate cancer should not lower their calorie intake. Also, you can break this rule on holidays—even as often as once a week when scheduling meals and other family logistics do not allow early meal times. Remember, having meals with people you love is also therapeutic, even if your dinnertime is later at night.

GOOD FISH

What To Do: Eat only "good" cold-water fish that is low in mercury, PCB's, and other toxic chemicals, and high in omega-3 fatty acids.

Why You Need It: Fish is one of nature's best anti-inflammatories. The reason: It's high levels of Omega-3 fatty acids. Cancer can become like a smoldering fire, which can slowly grow and spread. Anti-inflammatories like fish can keep those flames under control and even smother them. Research has linked fish consumption with a lower risk of prostate cancer death. (Chavarro et al. 2008) Another benefit of fish: selenium. This trace mineral serves as an antioxidant, which helps prevent cellular damage from free radicals. A meta-analysis of 20 studies showed a significant increase in the incidence of prostate cancer in men with low selenium levels.

Eat It: Wild Alaskan salmon, Atlantic Mackerel, and sardines. There are others detailed in the CaPLESS Food Rating System that are allowable.

When not to Eat it: If you are allergic to fish. Clearly, you need to abstain. Vegetarians and vegans do not need to eat fish to do well with the CaPLESS program, but do need to eat plenty of beans, flaxseeds, and whole grains. They supply sufficient protein and healthy fats to support your anticancer goals. Also, avoid(or at least eat very infrequently) swordfish, shark, tuna, snapper, grouper, king mackerel, marlin, and sea bass. These fish can be high in toxic mercury.

RAW NUTS AND SEEDS

What To Do: Nuts and seeds add flavor to all kinds of meals and also are great for snacks. Yes, they can be high in fat, which is why many men avoid them, but they have beneficial fat with many health benefits, they should become diet staples.

Why You Need It: Raw nuts and seeds are a traditional component of the Mediterranean Diet, which has been shown to have multiple health benefits including a top-notch cancer and heart disease fighter. Nuts are nutritional powerhouses because they are the source of a wide range of important nutrients, including proteins, unsaturated fatty acids, vitamins (B6, niacin, folic acid,), dietary fiber, copper, magnesium, potassium, zinc, antioxidants and many phytochemicals. In terms of cancer, nuts have shown some promise. For instance, a prospective trial of approximately 14,000 Seventh-day Adventist men showed an initial risk reduction of prostate cancer by 45 percent among those with higher nut consumption.

Eat It: The best nuts include walnuts, almonds, hazelnuts, pecans, cashews, and pistachios. The best seeds include pumpkin, sunflower, and flax seeds. You want to avoid salty and oil-roasted nuts. Stick with whole uncooked nuts with no added salt. Dry roasted are less protective but OK in a pinch.

When Not to Eat it: CaPLESS thrivers with kidney stones should stay away from nuts and seeds that are high in oxalates, like almonds and sesame seeds. Kidney stone sufferers should also drink plenty of water. There is some concern that nuts and seeds may pose a problem to patients with diverticulitis, as well. But the research is inconclusive, and the benefits of nuts and seeds may still outweigh the risk. You and your doctor can decide what makes the most sense for you.

HERBS AND SPICES

What To Do: Don't stop with a sprinkle here and a shake there. Add all kinds liberally to practically every meal.

Why You Need It: Looking for a true medical food? Herbs and spices have been used to treat illnesses since the days of ancient Egypt and Asia, and they are the foundation in Traditional Chinese Medicine and the Indian medical system Ayurveda. Herbs and spices have a strong reputation in the science world. They are one of the ultimate cancer fighters because they are full of powerful phytochemicals and antioxidants. And cancer hates these since they help drown the fire of inflammation and create a healthier environment for cells to thrive.

Eat it: There are so many to choose from, you are bound to find several you enjoy. These include: basil, sage, rosemary, turmeric, oregano, thyme, marjoram, ginger, cinnamon, cloves, coriander, cardamom, cumin, dill, saffron, allspice, etc. They are all 4s and 5s.

When Not to Eat: Some people are allergic to, or do not care for, spices like ginger, garlic, and turmeric. The benefits of those herbs do not out-weigh the discomfort. Also, some herbs and spices can trigger heartburn for people who suffer from acid reflux. The main heartburn offenders are the stronger spices: cloves, curry, nutmeg, mustard, and cayenne pepper.

Now you have a good sense of how to eat for maximal protection, and how easy it is to adopt and follow. Okay—maybe not that easy at first, but you will get there. Stick to it—CaPLESS eating can do so much for you.

Aside from helping to rid your body of built up additives, chemicals, and other junk, you are attacking your prostate cancer by feeding your body all the nutrients it needs to fight back. Along the way, you will no doubt lose weight, think clearer, and have more energy. Real food is *real* medicine.

Of course, eating well is one part of the program. The reality is that getting all the protective nutrients you need only from food is a challenge. Which brings us to the next pillar of the CM: incorporating the right kind of dietary supplements into your life

CM Profile: John, age 62

How CM worked: Taught him how to take charge to make change.

For John, CM Movement had the greatest impact on managing his prostate cancer. He choose active surveillance to monitor his low-risk cancer, but knew he need to change how he lived, especially when it came to exercise and fitness.

John's initial PSA at the age of 59, was 12.0ng/ml. He underwent a biopsy that revealed: 1 out of 12 cores positive, Gleason 7 (3+4). That was actually not as concerning to me as the fact that he was 6'3 and weighed 372 pounds. John was a walking time bomb, not from prostate cancer but from a heart attack. His blood lipid levels, which measure heart health were through the roof. He also complained of poor range of motion from his knees accompanied by a lot of knee pain. One year later he lost over one hundred pounds and decided to pursue Focal Ablation Therapy for his prostate cancer. He found that embracing the CM fitness taught him how to be more disciplined about his fitness and thus overall health.

He began a morning workout routine based on his current fitness level and grade of cancer . John chose a complete program he could easily do at home. He begins with neck and shoulder rolls as a warm up and then goes straight into a routine of 35 dumbbell push-ups and core work, then five minutes of 35-pound dumbbells moves for his biceps, triceps and back, followed by a series of squats and calf stretches. He then repeats the entire process three times and finishes on a stationary bike doing as many miles as in can in 10 minutes.

"It's short, and I don't have to find extra time in my schedule to do it," he says.

Best of all, he soon found the effects carried over into the rest of his day. "An early workout helps me make better decisions, and go to sleep earlier at night, so I feel fully rested, ready, and energetic for the next day and the next workout."

The new focus on regular movement also helped John adopt other aspects of the CM. "Each morning, as part of my postworkout routine, I have a protein shake with organic fruits and vegetables and pomegranate juice, which is an easy way to add many of the 4 and 5 foods into my diet," he says. "I also drink it with my first round of daily supplements, so I was able to take care of many parts of the program in one swoop."

Today, John's latest prostate biopsy shows no cancer in his prostate, he weighs 230 pounds, likely his normal weight for his body type and no aches and pain from his knees. His last PSA is 7.1ng/ml , still high but likely due to his large prostate which is still intact at 189 grams. Amazingly, he experience only minor urinary problems from his enlarged prostate.

CHAPTER 4

————— ⟨ ⟩ —————

A GUIDE TO DIETARY SUPPLEMENTS

Make it so no self-respecting cancer would ever want to inhabit your prostate.

—RONALD HOFFMAN, MD

No DIET IS perfect. No person is perfect. So it makes sense that even the most disciplined man will have trouble sticking to even an easy optimal eating program with no setbacks or slip-ups.

This is one of the main reasons I advocate daily supplementation as part of the CM arsenal. Supplements can ensure you fill any nutritional gaps and won't feel discouraged if you cannot follow CaPLESS eating all the time and everywhere you go.

When you think of supplements what is the first thing that comes to mind?

Generic multivitamins? Maybe a B-complex? You pop them even though you are not sure what they do and even if they are right for you. Unfortunately, this is a common issue with many people. There is supplementing, and there is what I call selected supplementation. By this I mean that you do not take supplements just to take them because they sound healthy, but rather focus only on the individual vitamins, minerals, and botanicals you specifically need to fight your prostate cancer and improve your overall health.

Selected supplementation does not involve grocery story one-a-days which are often stuffed with almost every type of vitamin and mineral available, some you need, some you don't, and with vast amounts that are not always ideal. Plus these types of multi-s typically are manufactured to include a list of others like dyes, colors, and unpronounceable words just like processed foods. Such dietary supplements are much like junk food.

You don't want to waste your time and money swallowing pills that are not designed to help you. Instead, you want to be smart, and focus on what you need and nothing else.

I cannot stress how essential I believe supplementation is for managing your prostate cancer. Besides supporting your CaPLESS eating to ensure you meet your daily nutritional needs, selected supplementation helps to build a huge arsenal in which to attack cancer cells and make your "biological soil" hostile to aberrations.

Selected supplementation is at the center of my naturopathic approach to medicine and wellness. There is much solid research along with my anecdotal evidence from patients illustrating that the right supplement combination is an integral part of overall wellness for men. Selected and judicious supplementation needs to be a regular part of every man's overall wellness and especially those who have or have had prostate cancer.

WHAT SUPPLEMENTS *CAN'T* DO

Don't fool yourself. Dietary supplements are not drugs or miracle workers that can cure a disease by themselves. Nor can they counteract the effects of a poor lifestyle filled with inadequate foods and little to no physical movement.

However, the judicious use of dietary supplements containing natural agents can assist in slowing or stopping cancer progression and development. The right type of supplements in the right combination and in the right amounts can support a healthy immune system, block pathways that promote prostate cancer, and reduce inflammatory markers that can influence cancer progression and promote overall health.

Over the years, though, dietary supplements have received a bad rap either through studies that question their effectiveness and safety or by deceptive claims from unscrupulous dietary supplement companies. On one end, poorly designed studies and bad hype have given supplements an undeserved black eye. On the other end, some dietary supplement facilities have either poor, noncompliant manufacturing practices or make unfounded claims that damage the reputation of all similar companies. This has caused many people to shy away from supplements even though they are often safe and potentially helpful.

The best example of the power of one bad study is the $170 million-plus Selenium and Vitamin E Cancer Prevention Trial, or the SELECT study. You may have read about it. The headlines proclaimed that taking selenium alone or in combination with vitamin E not only did not lower your risk of prostate cancer it actually could increase it.

Yet, one problem with the study was that it used only a single form of selenium (selenomethionine) and not the three different forms that were found protective against multiple cancers in high selenized yeast from SelenoExcell. If you think that is bad news, it gets worse. The study used only one form of vitamin E, a synthetic form known as dl-alpha tocopheryl acetate. Previous research has shown that when alpha tocopherol is taken by itself, it displaces gamma tocopherol—the form of vitamin E that is the most protective against prostate cancer and found in food.

So by supplementing aging men with only one form of vitamin E and one form of selenium, the SELECT scientists may have unwittingly increased subjects' prostate cancer risk by depriving prostate cells of essential critical gamma tocopherol, vitamin E, and the form selenium in high selenized yeast, SelenoExcell.

It may sound a bit confusing, but this is a classic example of how headlines and misleading information can tarnish the image of safe medicine. All you hear in the news is that vitamin E and selenium does not work for prostate cancer. Of course, not all stories on supplements are wrong as with the SELECT study, but it just solidifies how supplements can get an unfortunate negative image that may stick in the public's mind.

The bottom line: The right supplement combination has an important role in wellness, and is crucial to the CM. As long as you know what to take, how much, and what role they play in your prostate cancer management.

WHAT SUPPLEMENTS *CAN* DO

The right combination of supplements can help you live your best life after prostate cancer diagnosis. Selected supplementation works to address these five areas:

- boost immunity
- interrupt cancer formation
- reduce oxidative stress
- modulate inflammation
- improve detoxification

Boost Immunity. When it comes to fighting prostate cancer, your body's first defense is your immune system. And it begins with lymphocytes. These are part of what are called natural killer (NK) cells, which seeks out cancer cells and attacks them. NK cells hold the key to the growth and spread of prostate cancer.

NK cells are recognized as the immune system's front-line defense against cancer, viruses, and other pathogens like bacteria and parasites. Some research has indicated a strong link between pathogens and their ability to increase prostate cancer risk.

Interrupt Cancer Formation. Antitumor compounds work by directly and indirectly interfering with the body's ability to make cancer cells. Yet, cancer cells are smart and resourceful. In order for them to survive they need a steady stream of their own blood supply. As a result, they go through a mechanism of creating their own blood vessels (called angiogenesis) by producing a substance called vascular endothelial growth factor (VEGF).

Certain natural substances that I will discuss in a moment, like many found in some supplements, can block the action of VEGF, prevent the formation of blood vessels that surround and feed cancerous tumors, and therefore deprive them of nutrients they need to grow, thrive, and spread.

I am not saying dietary supplements serve as natural chemo. That has never been proven. What I am saying is that in nature there are agents that interfere with the pathways of the natural progression of cancer and when taken in proper amounts it can be *one* part of the anticancer arsenal. In fact, one of the most powerful chemo drugs, Docetaxel (generic), Taxotere (trade name) is derived from the bark of the Pacific yew tree.

Reduce Oxidative Stress. An antioxidant is a molecule that helps protect cells from the damaging effects of unstable molecules known as free radicals. Free radicals are released in the body from the detoxification system of your liver to fight toxins, such as artificial food colorings and flavorings, smog, preservatives in processed foods, alcohol, cigarette smoke, and pesticides. Some free radicals and reactive oxygen species (ROS) are needed for normal cellular function but often the amount of free radicals can overwhelm the body, causing what is called oxidative stress, and if left unchecked, can ignite bouts of inflammation that further fuels cancer growth.

However, feeding yourself with balanced antioxidants can eliminate free radicals and calm the storms of inflammation. Another method of boosting your body's antioxidant abilities is to stimulate the production of glutathione. Studies show that many cancer patients do not produce enough glutathione, which requires key nutrients like selenium and cysteine for its production.

Modulate Inflammation. Think of inflammation as a wild fire. When it gets out of control it can spread, grow, and consume everything around it. In your body, inflammation acts like fuel for your prostate cancer cells and makes them grow and spread at a faster rate. Research shows that this activity relies on the presence of the inflammatory marker that include Nuclear Factor Kappa B (NF-Kappa B), cyclooxygenase (COX and Interleukins (IL-6). Interfering with the production of these inflammatory chemicals make prostate cancer cells vulnerable and may reduce the formation and progression of cancer cells.

Improve Detoxification. Despite the digestive system's impressive function to keep bad stuff out of your body, some harmful substances can still make it to your blood stream, such as environmental carcinogenic compounds that promote prostate cancer, like cadmium, mercury, and xenoestrogens like BPA. So, your body needs the essential nutrients to further rid your system of toxins and remove procancer compounds.

Ultimately, it is your liver's responsibility to detect and rid the body of these unwanted substances. When the liver detects a toxic substance it breaks it down to become less harmful through a family of enzymes called cytochrome P450 (cP450). The goal of cP450 is to convert toxins into nontoxic substances that your body can get rid of through excretion. This is where supplements come into play. Specific nutrients help support this entire detox process and improve liver function to ensure it is successful.

A Note to Life Partner

You too can benefit from selected supplementation, so do not let it just be something he does alone. For example, women can benefit from the same omega-3 fatty acids and vitamin D supplements to provide basic nutrients for cancer protection and overall wellness. (For any of the other supplements highlighted here, consult with a nutritionally oriented physician.) So make supplements another daily ritual you do together. A tag team approach will also help to ensure that he does not forget to take his supplements, or have to be reminded all the time, which he will no doubt begin to resent because it will feel like you are constantly badgering him. This way you are both involved and can offer support for each other. If he considers taking supplements in lieu of living the CaPLESS lifestyle, gently nudge him back on track and remind him that the whole program is better than the sum of its parts.

NUTRIENTS SUPPORTED BY SCIENCE

Fourteen natural agents found in supplements are the core of the CM's selected supplementation program. They include the following:

- vitamin D
- Omega 3 fatty acids (fish oil)

- curcumin
- green tea extract
- grape seed extract
- selenium from high selenized yeast
- reishi mushroom
- pomegranate
- active hexose correlated compound (AHCC)
- modified citrus pectin (MCP)
- vitamin E
- zinc
- milk thistle
- broccoli extract (BroccoRaphanin)

As part of the CM's selected supplementation, you consider consuming all 14 ingredients in designated amounts and on a regular basis. Now, the number of supplements might sound daunting. After all, 14 is a rather high number and the idea of swallowing that many supplements every day can be overwhelming. But look at it this way: You are not just taking pills—but rather feeding your body what it needs to discourage aberrant cancer cells while boosting your health and wellness. Also, you will not have to take 14 separate pills each with the ingredients listed above. There are specialized formulas available that combine as many as eight of these ingredients into a single supplement.

Personally, I take many supplements every day and I have had patients who were once apprehensive about this approach, but they soon realized that it was no different than any other kind of daily health practice like exercising and brushing your teeth. I am confident you will feel the same, too.

However, if you do not feel comfortable taking multiple different supplements every day, there are formulas on the market that include many of these essential ingredients. They often are easier to take and manage. (See XYwellness.com at the resource page towards the end.)

Why are these specific supplements so special? Here is a detailed look at each one, how they might fight prostate cancer according to science, what the science says, and what is considered adequate daily amounts.

Vitamin D3

Why take it? Much research has linked vitamin D deficiency to many ill-nesses including type 2 diabetes, Alzheimer's disease, heart disease, and yes, most cancers, including prostate.

How much? 2,000–4,000 International Units (IUs) per day. More is often required in bigger people, but should only be taken under the supervision of a nutritionally oriented physician.

The Science A clinical trial used D supplementation at 4,000 IU per day for one year in men diagnosed with early stage, low-risk prostate cancer who were on active surveillance. Afterward, more than one-half showed a decreased number of positive prostate cores at a repeat biopsy.

Omega-3 fatty acids (fish oil)

Why take it? Fish oil comes from the tissue of fish and contains the omega-3 fatty acids known as eicosapentaenoic acid (EPA) and docosa-hexaenoic acid (DHA). EPA and DHA are known to reduce inflammation in the body and offer other health benefits.

How much? 2 to 4 grams per day.

The Science Much research has been conducted on the role of omega-3s to help with various health issues, including prostate cancer. For instance, researchers investigated the effect of dietary fish intake among 6,272 Swedish men over 30 years of age. The study reported that men who ate no fish had a two to three-fold increased risk for developing prostate cancer compared with those who consumed large amounts of fish in their diet.

Another study from the Harvard School of Public Health examined the link between dietary fish consumption and the risk of prostate cancer from spreading among 47,882 men. Over a 12-year period,

THRIVE DON'T ONLY SURVIVE

the researchers found that eating fish more than three times a week reduced the risk of prostate cancer, but had an even greater impact on the risk of metastatic prostate cancer.

For each additional 500 mg of fish oil consumed, the risk of metastatic cancer dropped by 24 percent. You may ask, "Why can't I just eat fish?" You can, of course. Fish is a regular part of CaPLESS eating, but it's not realistic to consume fish all the time, or in a high amount. Supplements are easy to take and help get the omega-3s you need.

CURCUMIN

Why take it? Curcumin is the active ingredient that gives the spice turmeric its rich fragrance and bright yellow-orange color. It has been used for centuries as a potent anti-inflammatory.

How much to take? 2,000 to 4,000 mg per day in divided doses.

The Science Chronic inflammation can cause all kinds of health problems in men from heart disease to certain cancers. In terms of prostate cancer, however, chronic inflammation elevates PSA in the prostate gland, which can built up and eventually leads to tumor formation. Curcumin is one of nature's most powerful anti-inflammatories.

If you have previously used or are currently under drug treatment or radiation for prostate cancer, research has suggested that the combination of curcumin with these common therapies could be an effective therapeutic approach for the treatment of prostate cancer, especially for men with drug or radiation resistance.

GREEN TEA EXTRACT

Why take it? Green tea contains high amounts of polyphenols, an antioxidant, which interferes with the activity of an enzyme called COX-2 that plays a key role in the development of prostate cancer.

How much to take? 300 mg of green tea extract two times a day.

The Science The relationship between green tea and prostate cancer has been well reached and the findings seem to point to one specific reaction: green tea slows the growth of prostate cancer cells and prompts them in essence to commit suicide. Green tea also encourages the repair of damaged DNA that might otherwise promote cancer growth.

GRAPE SEED EXTRACT (GSE)

Why take it? GSE is derived from the ground-up seeds of red wine grapes, so like grapes, it is rich in antioxidants, which soak up damaging free radicals in the body that can build up and promote cancer cell growth.

How much to take? 300 to 400 mg a day in divided doses.

The Science A 2011 study from the journal *Nutrition and Cancer* showed that GSE could reduce men's risk of prostate cancer by 40 to 60 percent. The research was conducted on 35,239 male participants in the Vitamins And Lifestyle (VITAL) study who were between the ages of 50 and 76. All participants were residents of Western Washington State and completed a detailed questionnaire about the 18 specialty supplements, as well as vitamin and mineral supplements, they were using or had used regularly over the past 10 years. Six years after the study's launch, the researchers found that men who regularly took GSE were 41 percent less likely to have been diagnosed with prostate cancer than a control group.

SELENIUM

Why take it? Selenium has shown to have some anticancer properties, lower blood pressure, contributes in glutathione production, and detoxifies the body of unwanted heavy metals like cadmium and mercury.

How much to take? 200 mcg per day of high selenized yeast, SelenoExcell. Never take more than 800 mcg of selenium a day

The Science The Nutritional Prevention Cancer (NPC) was Journal of American Medical Association (JAMA) published study to first show that high selenium yeast by SelenoExcell ® did not affect skin cancer incidence, but reduced the incidence of many cancers, especially prostate cancer by 63 percent. (Clark et al. 1996). On the Contrary, the SELECT study showed an increase in prostate cancer incidence when only selenomethionine was used, not the selenium enriched yeast used in the JAMA study by Clark et al. Lastly, a small recent study by a group of researchers at Penn State Medical University showed reduction in prostate cancer relevant biomarkers related to oxidative stress following supplementation with 285 mcg of selenium enriched yeast and not from selenomethionine. (Richie et al. 2014)

REISHI MUSHROOM
Why take it? Reishi, a popular medicinal mushroom, has been used in China for since ancient times to boost the immune system and fight infections. It also contains certain agents that have been shown to fight cancer tumors.

HOW MUCH TO TAKE? 500MG TO 1000MG PER DAY
The Science One study treated prostate cancer cells with 5 microl/ml reishi extract and discovered a 63.5 percent reduction in cell growth as well as a strong decrease in cell viability.

POMEGRANATE
Why take it? The pomegranate fruit has been used for centuries for medicinal purposes. The active ingredients of its juice are polyphenol punicalagins and ellagic acid, both having robust antioxidant properties.

How much to take? 200 to 225 mL (about 4 to 8 ounces) per day

The Science A clinical study found that the length of time it took for PSA levels to double after surgery or radiation was significantly longer in men who drank pomegranate juice. The subject had PSA levels of between 0.2 and 5 ng/mL and a Gleason score of 7 or higher. The results also found a 12 percent decrease in cell growth and a 17 percent increase in cell death.

ACTIVE HEXOSE CORRELATED COMPOUND (AHCC)

Why take it? AHCC is an extract derived from the *mycelia* of shiitake mushroom root threads. About 40 percent of AHCC is comprised of polysaccharides, which are known to have immune-stimulating effects. AHCC increases the production by immune cells of protein messengers. These proteins in turn promote the creation of macrophages, T cells, and NK cells to destroy cancerous cells.

How much to take? 1 to 3 grams per day.

The Science. AHCC studies are still ongoing, however, some clinical evidence indicates it may lower PSA levels and slow their growth. One study in the *Japanese Journal of Clinical Oncology* found that 55 percent of men who took AHCC supplements for six months were able to prolong their PSA doubling time to 120 months compared with only 39 percent who did not supplement.

MODIFIED CITRUS PECTIN (MCP)

Why take it? Pectins are especially concentrated in the peel and pulp of citrus fruits (lemons, limes, oranges, and grapefruits), as well as plums and apples. High levels of pectin are often used in jams and marmalades because of their gelling properties. Modified citrus pectin (MCP) is easily processed by the digestive system and absorbed into the bloodstream.

How much? 1,000 mg to 5,000 mg, two to three times a day.

The Science: Scientists believe MCP works by inhibiting two key processes involved in cancer progression: angiogenesis and metastasis. *Metastasis* occurs when cancer cells break away from the original tumor, enter the bloodstream or lymphatic system, and form a new tumor in a different part of the body.

Angiogenesis is when cancer cells make their own blood vessels to fuel their growth. In addition to its cancer-inhibiting effects, MCP shows promise in removing toxic heavy metals that can be so damaging to overall health.

VITAMIN E

What is it? Vitamin E is a group of nutrients in the form of tocopherols and tocotrienols, which best dissolve in fat. Each form has four types: alpha, beta, gamma, and delta. Gamma-tocopherol is the most abundant form found in food. **Why take it?** Both forms, tocopherol and tocotrienols, seem to have protective qualities against prostate cancer and heart disease most likely due to its strong antioxidant capacity.

How much to take? 100 to 400 International Units (IU) of mixed tocopherols and higher gamma-tocopherols—but *never* just alpha-tocopherol. Do not take more than 50 IU of synthetic alpha-tocopherol, if at all. Sometimes this is the form found in many formulas.

The Science One study from Johns Hopkins looked at more than 10,000 men and found that those with the highest blood levels of gamma-tocopherol concentrations had a five-fold lower risk of prostate cancer compared with men in the lowest quintile. This effect was not significant for plasma alpha-tocopherol concentrations.

ZINC

What is it? Zinc is essential for life. Oysters contain more zinc per serving than any other food, but red meat and poultry provide the majority of zinc in the Western diet. Numerous experimental studies have provided compelling evidence that zinc has a protective effect against prostate carcinogenesis.

Why take it? Zinc has many healthy properties including strengthening the immune system. This mineral is second only to iron in terms of its concentration in the body and it works together with more than 300 enzymes in three major biological roles: structural, regulatory, and as catalyst. Concentration in prostate tissue is dependent on the aggressiveness of prostate cancer—the higher the Gleason score, the greater the local zinc depletion.

How much to take? 15 mg to 30 mg a day. More than 100 mg a day for a prolonged period of time actually may promote prostate cancer.

The Science: The normal human prostate contains one of the highest amounts of zinc in the body. Zinc continuously decreases in the prostate in early to late cancer cells. In one study, long-term supplemental zinc intake was associated with reduced risk of advanced and potentially deadly prostate cancer.

Milk Thistle
What is it? Milk Thistle is an herb that contains a protective molecule called silibinin.

Why take it? It promotes antiangiogenesis, protects the liver and supports liver detoxification, and reduces proinflammatory chemicals.

How much to take? 100 to 200 mg a day

The Science One clinical trial involving adult men with prostate cancer reported delays in rising prostate specific antigen levels compared with a placebo group. Again, the key ingredient in milk thistle appears to be silibinin. It has been shown to possess antioxidant effects and protect against depletion of glutathione, one of the liver's most important antioxidants.

BROCCOLI SEED EXTRACT (BROCCORAPHANIN)
What is it? Broccoli seeds are particularly rich in sulforaphane glucosinolate (SGS), which is needed to make a protective chemical called sulforaphane.

Why take it? Since sulforaphane was identified in 1992 by researchers at the Johns Hopkins University School of Medicine, there have been hundreds of studies demonstrating its protective benefits, including a reduced risk of many cancers and enhancing phase-two 2 detoxification (see page 146 on detoxification). Keep in mind that sulforaphane is not found in broccoli, but rather made from SGS in broccoli.

How much to take? 100 to 500 mg per day

The Science: Sulphoraphane has shown to induce death of aggressive prostate cancer cells in test tubes, and reduce spreading of such malignant cells in animal models. One human study showed significant prostate cancer protection in a group of men who consumed 400 mg of broccoli a week compared to another group consuming 400 mg of peas a week.

Remember: The judicious and careful use of dietary supplements is only one part of the overall arsenal against prostate cancer. It does not replace the other crucial elements of the CM. Dietary supplements are not wonder drugs, but the right combination play a vital role in creating an inhospitable environment for cancer. If you already take supplements of some kind this will be easier to embrace, but if the act of taking daily pills is new, don't fret. Just like any other aspect of improving your health and wellness, it is only new at the beginning. As you progress and become more comfortable with the daily habit of ingesting supplements, you will see them as just another part of your new, healthy, and vibrant life.

BLENDS AND FORMULAS WORTH CONSIDERING

With few exceptions, dietary supplements do not come as single agents in a bottle. The aforementioned ingredients are typically found in many synergistic blends. However, if you are more comfortable taking formulas and blends (and thus less pills per day), here are some choices that I have clinically used and are worth trying:

IMMUNOPCTN®

What is it? A blend of grape seed extract, boswelia, curcumin, pomegranate extract, reishi mushroom, green tea extract, and modified citrus pectin.

Why take it? I formulated ImmunoPCTN with the idea of having the most science-based, cancer protective ingredients in a single bottle. All the individual ingredients are backed up by hundreds of studies that support improved immunity and anti-inflammatory benefits. Also, modified citrus pectin has shown to stabilize PSA, rid the body of cadmium and mercury, and inhibit unwanted Galectin-3, which is a molecule involved in spreading cancer.

How much to take? three pills, two times a day, without food

ZYFLAMEND

What is it?: Zyflamend is a dietary supplement that contains extracts of rosemary, turmeric, ginger, holy basil, green tea, hu zhang, Chinese goldthread, barberry, oregano, and Baikal skullcap.

Why take it?: Zyflamend has been shown to have anti-inflammatory effects via inhibition of cyclooxygenase (COX) activity. COXs are enzymes that convert arachidonic acid into prostaglandins, which are thought to play a role in tumor development and growth. One COX enzyme, COX-2, is activated during chronic disease states, such as cancer.

How much to take? Take three to four pills a day in divided doses.

POMI-T

What is it? A dietary supplement formula consisting of broccoli powder, turmeric powder, pomegranate, green tea 5:1 extract (20 mg equivalent to 100 mg of green tea).

Why take it? Pomi-T, made by Nature Medical in the United Kingdom, has many of the listed ingredients that show protection against cancer cells. In one study there seemed to be a decrease in prostate cancer progression along with PSA stabilization.

How much to take? one pill, three times a day

GDTOXSEL®
What is it? It is a blend of botanicals and nutrients including selenium (SelenoExcell), reduced glutathione, vitamin E (mixed tocopherols, higher gamma tocopherol), zinc, vitamin C, alpha lipoic acid, milk thistle, broccoli extract (broccoraphnine), schisandra berry extract.

Why take it? It is a great blend of balanced antioxidants with nutrients that assist in phase 1 and phase 2 detoxification.

How much to take? 3 pills a day in divided doses.

CM Profile: Samuel, age 67

How did CM help: Showed how to generate positive change when you are on active surveillance.

Samuel was not your typical prostate cancer patient. He was a trim and fit retiree with low-risk cancer. When I met Sam in July 2013 he was 66 years old with a PSA was 5.04ng/ml. His prostate biopsy revealed: Two positive cores with Gleason scores of 6. Sam was nervous about his prostate cancer situation and began to make sure his affairs were in order. He thought he was done. His Medical team and I did not only think he would overcome prostate cancer but also concluded that he would be the perfect candidate for no aggressive treatment. Sam began on an Active surveillance (or as I call, ProActive Surveillance), and he avoided what he felt were stressful treatments in exchange for being closely monitored by his medical team.

But he did not want to do nothing about his condition. "Odds are that I'm going to die from something else and not the prostate cancer," he says. "Still, it did make me take a closer look at my overall health to see what I could be doing to make sure the cancer stays nonthreatening," he says.

Two areas of the CM that helped Samuel the most were the addition of supplements and mind-body practices.

He found that following the supplements program gave him increased energy and helped to increase vital nutrients that were lacking in his usual diet. Daily meditation, mantra recitals, and regular yoga have refocused his outlook on his condition so he is more positive and optimistic about his future. "I feel I have cured my cancer. I believe that and I live like that," he says.

He continues to get his PSA tested every three months, and so far, not only has it not gone up, but has even dropped some. "So what I'm doing now must be working," he says.

Today Sam is a vibrant extraordinary fit almost 70 years-old with PSA of 4.3, no evidence of cancer progression and enjoying life with his son and grandkids with extraordinary health. Sam is now engaged to a lovely woman.

CHAPTER 5

MOVEMENT

Lack of activity destroys the good condition of every human being, while movement and methodical physical exercise save it and preserve it.

—Plato (427–347 BC)

LET ME GET right to the point. If you really want to live your best life, you need to be physically active, doing both high and low intensity movement, every day, for the rest of your life. Plain and simple. The only way to live longer, better, and healthier is to develop a strong body. Regular movement, combined with high and low intensity, is an essential component for the CM, and getting and staying out of your comfort zone is necessary to staying physically active.

The good news is you do not need to spend two or three hours in the gym or pounding away on the treadmill. You only need the Lowest Effective Dose, or what I call, LED, which is the least amount of work you need to do get maximal results. For my program, the LED is three hours per week with moderate to high intensity. No less. Of course, more is always good, but do not do more than six hours a week of moderate to high intensity exercise.

You cannot take it easy during your workouts either. You have to work hard and be consistent. You need to challenge yourself to build up muscle and a good sweat.

Let me to be clear: fitness is instrumental in your overall health and wellness and a must for prostate cancer management and recurrence prevention. I'm emphasizing this fundamental point because some of you may resist exercising consistently with the "I don't have time" excuse. You can follow everything else in the CM, but if you fail to embrace movement and fitness at the level and intensity you need, you will not live your best life. The research on this is clear, and I will help you implement it regardless of your current level of fitness or the stage of your prostate cancer. No excuses.

Now I know you might find exercising less than a pleasant experience. OK, let's be honest, you may downright hate it. But even if you were a high school nerd or were never picked for a street ball game, you can find a movement prescription that's right for you. No success comes easy. But after clinically seeing thousands of prostate cancer patients adopt the movement part of the CM, I can tell you that this part of the program is critical.

I know you are busy and perhaps a little older with some extra flab around your waist. You are not as active as you once were, and it's harder to get motivated to exercise, and no doubt harder on your body—even physically and mentally painful at times.

I'm right up there with you. Personally, I don't have a problem getting up early to go for a run or to the gym most of the time. Other times it takes a whole lot of effort and will power—a lot of will power. My problem is scheduling my workouts in since I have so much to do. But in the end, my busy schedule does not matter as much as living a great life. What is your motivation? What is your why? Your why is the driving force to get you going.

What matters is that I live my best life—and that you live your best life too, so you can spend great times with your friends, family, kids, and grandkids. That's what it is all about. And it takes work. There are no free lunches and no excuses. You and your family deserve the very best from you. Don't you think?

You hate exercise? So do I, as does almost everyone else I meet. But believe me, it will grow on you. Once you begin to feel strong and see the results, you will be motivated to exercise consistently. You may never love it, but that's fine. You will do it anyway simply because you want to live your best life, and you know from years of experience that nothing worthwhile ever comes easy.

A Note to Your Life Partner

With time, regular movement will make him feel energetic and strong. I have had couples that choose to work out together almost every day. My advice: share a fitness goal like running a 5K. Goals are important for men to stay consistent with a training regimen. One of my prostate cancer patients likes to exercise by himself, but enjoys tango dancing with his wife once or twice a week. Another patient really enjoys working out with his wife. "It is another way for us to spend quality time together," he says. Figure what works best for you—and him—and go from there.

Don't be surprised if you see a spike in your sex life as you both become more active. I'm not kidding. Sweaty hands, racing pulse, and shortness of breath all ignite physical attraction. Plus, regular exercise also may help avoid some common prostate cancer treatment side effects, even sexual dysfunction. A 2013 study involving 57 men on androgen suppression therapy for prostate cancer found that those who exercised twice weekly for 12 weeks increased both their sexual interest and activity. Those in the control group who did not exercise found their sexual life decreased over the same period. iii So exercise is good for you, him, and your life as a couple.

THE SCIENCE OF EXERCISE AND PROSTATE CANCER

You may already be familiar with many of the common benefits of regular exercise—lower stress, weight loss, better sleep, and a bunch of other advantages. Research has shown that fitness can help you reduce your risk of developing prostate cancer, prevent it from returning, or lower the chances of you dying from it.

Also, you can overcome common side effects from treatments, and even lower your risk of dying from other causes. Don't forget—while prostate cancer can indeed be deadly, many men with prostate cancer pass away from something else, but live the rest of their life in constant worry about their PSA levels.

Remember, it is not only about how many years you live, but also how you live those years. Here is a look at the key reasons exercise is so crucial for fighting prostate cancer.

1. IMPROVE INSULIN SENSITIVITY

For starters, exercise helps to improve insulin sensitivity. When you engage in intense exercise, your muscles gobble up excess sugar in your bloodstream for energy without the need for extra insulin produced by the pancreas. With less insulin, and thus less sugar-energy, cancer cells are deprived of the fuel they demand. A big part of creating an environment hostile to cancer is starving cancer cells of their energy. So every time you engage in high-intensity exercise, you help to kill cancer cells by starving them of sugar.

2. IMPROVES THE FUNCTION OF YOUR SEWAGE SYSTEM

Regular exercise also improves the function of your lymphatic system, which is a complex network of organs, lymph nodes, lymph ducts, and lymph vessels that make and move lymph fluid from tissues to the bloodstream.   The lymph fluid is filled with your body's army of white blood cells and works by taking your "dirty" blood, sending it through the lymphatic system for "cleaning," then returning "clean" fluid back into the circulatory system. Keeping your lymphatic system clean is yet another means to create the thriving healthy environment that is hostile to cancer cells.

There are two main ways to improve the movement of your lymphatic system: deep breathing and muscle contraction. As you huff and puff and muscles tighten, lymph vessels are squeezed—like milking a cow—and your body's junk in the lymph fluid is pushed along, filtered through lymph nodes bringing back clean fluid to the veins and the heart. It is important to keep the lymph fluid moving smoothly in order to efficiently move out waste, and working your muscles is the best way to do that.

3. KEEP YOUR BODY WEIGHT LOW

Exercise also helps maintain a healthy weight and keeps your body fat low, both of which can reduce your chances of prostate cancer recurrence and lowers your risk of dying from prostate cancer. Increasing evidence suggests that obesity (either before or at the time of diagnosis) is strongly associated with prostate cancer progression and prostate cancer-specific mortality. A 2011 study among 2,546 men diagnosed with localized prostate cancer found that a one-unit increase in body mass index (BMI) was associated with an approximately 10 percent increase in the risk of prostate cancer death, and BMI of at least 30 kg/m2 was associated with a nearly twofold increased risk. Keep your weight under control and you can better beat prostate cancer for good.

Time and effort are at the center of the CaPLESS Movement. You need to commit to both to be successful. An easy way to incorporate regular exercise into your life is to schedule it like you do so many other events. Be serious about your fitness. Put it into your daily calendar like you would schedule a business lunch or meeting with your most important client. Commit to it as though you would a meeting with your boss when you are up for a 20 percent raise. You would not think of blowing off those appointments, would you? Give your training the same respect. If you want to live your best life, you have to respect your body and give it the attention it needs—every day.

THE RIGHT AMOUNT OF TIME

Now here's the kicker. You have to put in the time to receive the benefits. It is simple math. Devote proper time to fitness and you can reduce your cancer risk and live your best life.

How much exercise is enough and what is your LED? A recent study found that among 2,705 men with localized prostate cancer, which had not spread, those who engaged in three hours or more of vigorous physical activity per week had a 49 percent lower risk of death from all causes and a 61 percent reduced risk of dying from prostate cancer, compared with men who got less than one hour of vigorous activity per week.[i]

Only vigorous exercise was associated with a reduced risk of death from prostate cancer. The findings suggest that if you have prostate cancer, engaging in at least three hours a week of vigorous exercise may improve your chances of surviving the disease. Those three hours can be broken down anywhere from 30 minutes daily for six days to an hour a day for three days per week. More is OK and even encouraged as you become more comfortable and are inspired by the results.

But your LED is only four hours a week. That is nothing. You have that time in your life. I don't care how busy you think you are. Think about the small things you do every day that easily add up to three hours: watching TV, returning e-mails that can wait. You have the time. Use it well!

LED AND INTENSITY

Physicians suggest that some movement is better than nothing. I agree. If you are stuck at zero and move into the positive, this is good. But to really address your prostate cancer and significantly improve your longevity, low intensity movement will only help to a point. You need to crank it up eventually. No rush. Progress when you are ready. But at least keep up a moderate intensity during those three hours of your LED to live your best life.

Exercise should be a lifetime journey. It is increasingly clear that low intensity exercise only does so much in terms of insulin resistance, reducing inflammation, or shrinking body fat. In other words, a casual stroll through the mall or slow walk on the treadmill while holding on to the bar is a good start if you are not used to exercising. I applaud if you have taken those steps to moving forward. I know even this amount may not be easy for some of you.

At some point you need to upgrade from the mall and turn up the speed and elevation on the treadmill. Don't blame me—I'm just the messenger. This is what the science shows. It's pretty clear.

In fact, in one-study, researchers found that brisk walking (at slight fast pace) three hours per week was associated with a lower recurrence of progression compared with walking at an easier pace for the same time period.[ii]

That's good, right? Yes and no. Yes, brisk walking is better than a lower intensity stroll, but the researchers found that when you turn up the dial and make walking a real aerobic effort—or even jump into higher intensity activities like running or cycling—the benefits become bigger.

So how can you determine how much intensity is enough? There are easy two ways: The Talk Test and the Heart Rate Monitor.

The Talk Test This is an easy and subjective method to measure how hard you work during exercise. Moderate intensity exercise is when you can comfortably carry conversation with someone, but cannot sing (for comparison, with low intensity you can sing). With high intensity you should only be able to say three or four words at a time, but not be able to complete a sentence. This is easy to do during any type of exercise to constantly remind yourself to turn up the intensity when needed.

Heart Rate Monitor (HRM) This device, which resembles a wristwatch, measures your heartbeats per minute. Using this measurement, slow-intensity exercise is defined as a level of activity that raises the heart rate to about 30 percent to 50 percent of your maximum heart rate. (See sidebar for a list of maximum heart rates based on age.) Examples of low-intensity activities include walking at a rate of two to three miles per hour or bicycling at a 10 miles per hour pace.

Moderate exercise is defined as activity carried out at 55 to 70 percent of maximum heart rate. Examples include walking at three miles per hour or bicycling at 10 to 20 miles per hour.

Vigorous exercise is defined as requiring 70 to 95 percent of maximum heart rate. This is the range you want to aim for in order to receive the greatest benefits. Running at 5 miles per hour or faster, or bicycling at a speed higher than 20 miles per hour, would be considered vigorous activity. (Note: if you are in really good shape, you can run at 5 miles an hour and not raise your heart rate to 70 percent maximum, so you will have to turn up the intensity.)

Find Your Maximum Heart Rate

Your maximum heart rate is about 220 minus your age. As you exercise, you want to periodically monitor your heart rate to ensure you stay within the appropriate range to maintain vigorous exercise. You can do this with a heart-rate monitor or you can measure it manually.

• *Take your pulse on the inside of your wrist, on the thumb side.*

• *Use the tips of your first two fingers (not your thumb) to press lightly over the blood vessels on your wrist.*

• *Count your pulse for 10 seconds and multiply by 6 to find your beats per minute.*

Age	HR Zone 50–85 percent	Average Maximum Heart Rate, 100 percent
40 years	90–153 beats per	180 beats per minute
45 years	88–149 beats per minute	175 beats per minute
50 years	85–145 beats per minute	170 beats per minute
55 years	83–143 beats per	165 beats per minute
60 years	80–136 beats per minute	160 beats per minute
65 years	78–132 beats per minute	155 beats per minute
70 years	75–128 beats per minute	150 beats per minute

CAPLESS MOVEMENT BEYOND EXERCISE

Now that you are committed to exercise as a lifestyle (and you *are* committed, aren't you?) I have some good more news. In order to live your best life, prevent another cancer diagnosis, or possible heart attack, you have to remain as active as possible even after workouts.

In other words, even after you apply your LED movement plan, or after you go beyond your LED, sitting around for more than two hours at a time can still increase your risk of premature death from cancer or heart disease. In other words, the chair is deadly. We simply have not evolved to sit around much. Thousands of years ago, if you sat around too much, you were eaten for lunch. Clearly we don't have saber tooth tigers chasing us anymore, but the outcome can be the same if you stay immobile for too long. Modern day work life has made continuous movement almost impossible, I know. How can you keep today's saber tooth from eating you? Here's what you can do:

- Set your smartphone or computer alarm to every 50 minutes and go for a 5-to-10 minute walk. It can be in your office, but outside in the fresh air and sunshine would be better.
- Skip the elevator and take the stairs.
- If your budget and work environment allow, get a treadmill desk, which lets you read, write, and work on a computer while walking at a slow, but steady pace.
- Get an elevated desk with a stool where you can alternate standing and sitting.
- Conduct phone conferences standing.

THE RIGHT CAPLESS MOVEMENT PROGRAM FOR YOU

Duration and intensity are keys for optimal exercise, but does it matter what you do? Not really. You need to work hard with the right intensity, blood pumping, and your muscles activated. What allows you to reach that intensity level really depends on your current health status and fitness level.

Power walking can make you really sweat if you are overweight and new to exercise. Others may need to hit the treadmill at a good speed and pace. Then there are men who can get their cardiovascular system going by lifting weights, while others work out their muscles from a good yoga routine.

Mix it up. Work up a sweat. Stay moving.

CaPLESS movement is not about doing specific exercises. Instead, it helps you find the right combination of fitness you need and at the right intensity. However, you do not want to just focus on one activity—say running—all the time and not do anything else. Running is a great form of exercise, gets you sweating, and engages many muscles, but it has its limits. You need an all-around exercise program that combines the three main components for optimal fitness: aerobic, strength training, and stretching.

It is difficult, if not impossible to create broad-based exercise plans that are ideal for everyone. However, it is possible to design an individualized program covering these areas. CaPLESS movement does this based on a simple formula that takes into account three criteria:

1. Prostate cancer diagnosis (its stage and aggressiveness)
2. Current treatment (i.e., active surveillance, hormone therapy, surgery)
3. Current fitness level (ranging from zero to three, from not that active to exercising on a regular basis)

This mix-and-match approach helps to addresses your present needs while helping you adopt the kind of vigorous exercise you need to better manage your prostate cancer and overall health and wellness. For more specific guidance go to www.ThriveDontOnlySurvive.com to create your own individualized CaPLESS movement program. Each workout will outline how to reach the level of needed intensity in terms of duration, resistance, and time (for aerobics), repetitions, sets, and desired weights (for strength training), and stretching sequence. Also, you will find workouts for your specific situation; for example, while on hormone therapy.

You will also be given a sample week-long plan to follow as well as alternative exercises so you can switch out workouts as needed without having to worry about losing momentum, motivation, or interest. This way you can be assured to find something you enjoy doing.

CM Profile: William (better known as Bill)

How CM Helped: CM Movement soothed the side effects of radiation therapy.

Bill, 83, and his physician, made the decision to use hormone depletion therapy to help with his prostate cancer. He received a Lupron injection every three months and underwent 43 radiation treatments over a nine-week period. While this helped his prostate cancer, his health suffered. After a year, his testosterone levels were near zero and he experienced severe muscles loss and weakness.

He turned to the CM Movement to rebuild his strength and embrace the supplement regime to boost his nutritional needs. He also needed help with common side effects like urinary incontinence and night sweats. "The night sweats were terrible," he says. "It would be so bad I had to change my PJs several times a night."

He did CM Movement exercises with a trainer three days a week. As part of the program, he focused on strengthening his pelvic floor muscles, which helped to control his urinary incontinence. "Most men don't even know where these muscle are, let alone how to engage them."

Core muscle training built up his lost strength. "When I began, I could barely lift a five-pound weight. Now I am up to 20 pounds," he says.

His regular routine also included four miles on the treadmill, 10 minutes of rowing, and multiple sets of free weights. Bill also adopted controlled breathing techniques to help with the mental stress of treatments. When he was not in the gym, he used every opportunity to squeeze in some kind of exercise, like skipping the elevator for the stairs.

As a result, he was able to manage and in some cases eliminate all the side effects. No more night sweats. No more muscle weakness. No more bathroom issues. Along the way he discovered the CM Movement influenced other parts of his life. "I was sleeping well and waking at seven a.m. ready for a full day," Bill says.

"It is amazing how quickly the body reacts when you give it a chance."

CHAPTER 6

STRESS AND SLEEP

Sleep is the chief nourisher in life's feast.

—William Shakespeare

We talk a lot about stress, but what is it exactly? Stress can come from internal or external factors. For example, a thought or a feeling can cause a stressful reaction, or the response may be triggered from an external source like a loud noise. There's also physical stress, which can be a good thing—like during high intensity exercise. There is also psychological stress during an argument with your spouse, or battling coworkers.

No matter the cause, stress manifests in your body in the same way: Your body launches a fight-or-flight response, releasing stress chemicals to help protect you from the taxing encounter. Thousands of years ago, this biological stress response enabled humans to escape from dangerous situations (like, say, a saber-toothed tiger that wants you for dinner). But while our day-to-day lives have greatly evolved since then, our stress responses haven't.

As a result, modern men live half their lives on "high alert" due to much more mundane daily triggers, like traffic jams, demanding jobs, or financial worries. And while good in short spurts, this kind of excess stress can be damaging. Stress is a pivotal player in managing your condition. I have found that the type of stress that has the most significant impact on your postdiagnosis health is psychological stress.

THE BRIEF SCIENCE OF STRESS

Anything that poses the perception of a threat to our well-being causes stress. But here's the deal: You need stress in your life. Without it, you would not survive. It is not a matter of stress as good or bad, but rather that an excess of anything can be detrimental to your post cancer health.

When you participate in exercise and movement, for example, you stress your body so it can grow and become stronger. Stressing your muscles is absolutely essential to make them stronger. That is good stress. If someone is threatening your life chasing you with a knife, you will have to either fight or flee. Your body produces stress chemicals called cortisol, epinephrine, and norepinephrine to help you escape danger.

Suddenly, your blood pressure rises, breathing becomes more rapid, your digestive system slows down to conserve energy, and you experience a heightened state of alertness—all good things needed in an attempt to survive.

While these stress chemicals serve you well in time of danger, chronic production, especially cortisol, can weaken your immune system to the point where a favorable cancer environment is created.

To bring it even closer to home, stress can be such a powerful entity that it affects the accuracy of your PSA scores. One study examined 1,600 men to look at the effect of stress on PSA, and showed that prostate cancer-specific worry was linked with significantly abnormal PSA level when perceived cancer risk, cancer worry, and cancer-related symptoms were present. That's why physicians often jokingly say PSA stands for Patient Stimulated Anxiety.

STRESS AND YOUR IMMUNE SYSTEM

You immune system kicks in when something invades your body: a virus, bacteria, or formation of a cancer cell, etc. It behooves you to maintain a strong immune system at all times. If not, uninvited visitors would have a feast.

Your immune system is tightly connected to your psyche. What you think has an impact on your immune system. Good thoughts strengthens your immunity while bad thoughts weakens it.

For instance, chronic, uncontrolled stress suppresses your immune system from overproduction of cortisol. Cortisol influences most cells that participate in the immune reaction, especially white blood cells, but also the natural killer cells, monocytes, macrophages, and mast cells. These cells are important because they should be awake, strong, and on patrol—ready to fight cancerous cells and protect you.

WHAT YOU CAN DO NOW

ADAPT TO CHANGE

Nothing is permanent and change is inevitable. Stressful events will occur—that's life. The goal here is not to protect yourself from all stress, but simply to modify your perspective, so when you are faced with stress you can better manage it—instead of it managing you.

When you can better control your reaction to stressful events, you can keep the damaging chemicals from being over produced and thus promoting cancer development and progression. Try some of these techniques:

CONTROL YOUR MONKEY MIND

Monkey mind is a term for an unsettled, uncontrollable, and indecisive mind—like monkeys, jumping, screeching, chattering, and carrying on endlessly. Learn to calm your monkey mind when negative thoughts arise by doing focused deep breathing. Practice daily for 10 minutes a day so when the monkeys begin their havoc you can counter with several rounds of deep breathing. (See Sidebar.)

DON'T MAKE UP YOUR OWN STORIES

In other words, don't create false realities that make you feel like crap. Most of the times, it is not the truth that stresses you, but your interpretation of the truth. For example, rising PSA after medical treatment for prostate cancer does not always equal death. In fact, it often doesn't. So don't think along those lines if you are in that situation and ask your physician what results and changes really mean before you jump to conclusions.

Prostate cancer is a different beast altogether when compared to other cancers—pancreatic, for example. Let your doctor explain to you what the numbers *really* mean—most of the time it is not a morbid situation. At the same time, don't create false realities that make you feel temporarily good about yourself. It is a mistake to think you are completely home free after prostate cancer treatment and that you don't need to follow a lifestyle program that protects you like the CaPLESS Method. The recurrence rate after cancer treatment is more than 35 percent. Most importantly, the prostate is (or was if surgically removed) not separate from your body. Your body is all connected. If your prostate had cancer, where else are cancer cells harboring?

LIVE YOUR LIFE ON PAPER

Write down your thoughts on paper. This means everything from buying flowers for your wife on your anniversary to meeting with my accountant on May 20 at 12:30 p.m. at his office. Sometimes stress can result from having too much in your head and fear that you may forget something. Also, writing down things de-clutters your head and will bring you clarity for handling the people and events that have a higher importance in your life. Get a little pocket-size notebook to carry with you at all times. I can't live without my little red moleskin notebook myself. Of course, if you are a techy, you can type everything in your smart phone. I actually use both. Anything to free up my mind.

HAVE REALISTIC EXPECTATIONS

You will have challenges in life. It is part of being alive. Life crises are also part of living. Bestselling self-improvement author Brian Tracy says, "You are either in a crisis now, just came out of one, or will be in one soon." Thinking that everything is going to be a bed of roses all the time is unrealistic. So is the idea that there is doom around every corner. Embrace the fact that there are regular ups and downs and sometimes the downs are steep. The benefit here is simple acknowledgment that some crisis will happen at some point, and this mind-set prepares you to better deal when it arrives.

EXERCISE

Frequent physical exercise is not only an integral part of the CM, but it is also a major stress buster that forces you to breathe deeply and produce feel-good chemicals (dopamine and endorphins), and it helps you get good sleep. There is also strong evidence that physically fit people have less extreme physiological responses when under pressure. This means that fitter people are more able to handle the long-term effects of stress, without suffering from health problems or burnout. So get moving now.

THINK POSITIVE

Why do the things that drive you mad never bother some people? Take a lesson from Buddhists and strive to see everything as stress-less, and not stressful. The idea is that objects cannot be stressful all by themselves— you have to interpret them that way. Which is better: cursing rose bushes for having thorns—or celebrating the fact thorn bushes have roses. It is your choice. I am not saying to think," there are no weeds in your lawn," when there are. As bestselling author and life strategist Anthony Robbins would say, "If there are weeds, go take them out."

LAUGH

This is one of the quickest stress-busters. It counteracts cortisol (remember too much cortisol from stress is no good) and it allows your brain to learn and think about new and less stressful things. When you're serious, you're most likely in a protection mode—only solving old problems, not creating a new future. Read funny jokes. Find funny people. Watch funny videos on YouTube. Laugh all the way to the bank.

MANAGE YOUR FINANCES INTELLIGENTLY

Don't take on more financial responsibilities, such as a new car or a bigger house, if you think they'll be a stretch. Being realistic about your finances is an important strategy for managing stress. Live way under your means, and be careful not to go shopping to cope with stress rather than getting things that you need. As Bruce Lee said, "The more we value things, the less we value ourselves."

RESOLVE ISSUES BEFORE THEY BECOME CRISES

It's human nature to avoid unpleasant topics and circumstances, but if you're concerned about a brewing situation, whether it's at work or at home, address it early to keep it from becoming more serious, harder to solve, and more stressful for you. Problems are always easier to handle before they develop into full-blown calamities.

TAKE A TIME OUT

Daily stressors can creep up on you before you realize it, so treat yourself to at least one relaxing activity every day. Listen to music, meditate, write in a journal, or enjoy a soothing bath are all great ways to relax and relieve stress. Taking time for yourself is important for both preventing and managing stress.

SLEEP AND PROSTATE CANCER

This brings me to what I believe is the number-one stressor for most men: lack of proper sleep. The average amount of sleep has consistently declined and deteriorated since the advent of modern technology. Texting, emailing, or watching the tube can be a sleep killer. Work stress, an unstable economy, and health problems do not help.

An occasional sleepless night usually isn't much of a problem, but running a sleep deficit over time can cause serious issues. Every system in your body is affected by lack of sleep. Restorative sleep is an essential ingredient for a healthy mind and body.

However, hypercompetitive men and much of Western society in general think sleep is a waste of time and a luxury for the lazy. The notion that successful people can get by with just a few hours of sleep a night without paying the price is not only erroneous, but dangerous.

There is nothing wrong with being competitive or successful, or course—both can be healthy. But when sleep is consistently sacrificed to obtain a competitive edge, due to stress or any other reason, you will damage your long-term health and promote prostate cancer. In the end you may not be successful either.

Sleep Apnea

If you suffer from sleep apnea, you have a higher risk of cancer, according to recent research. Sleep apnea is a common sleep disorder that affects up to 7 percent of men. It involves repetitive episodes of complete or partial upper airway obstruction occurring during sleep despite an ongoing effort to breathe. Common symptoms include snoring, fatigue, and dangerous pauses in breathing at night. A recent study in the Journal of Clinical Sleep Medicine found that cancer mortality was 3.4 times more common in those with sleep apnea than with no sleep apnea, among 5,200 people who were followed for 20 years. The researchers found that the greater the extent of hypoxemia, or oxygen depletion, during sleep, the more likely a person would receive a cancer diagnosis. If you believe you may suffer from sleep apnea, see your doctor and schedule a visit to a sleep clinic.

WHY IS SLEEP IMPORTANT?

There are two main hormones that are affected by poor quality sleep: melatonin and cortisol.

Melatonin is a powerful antioxidant that helps the body suppress the production of estrogen—a possible contributor to prostate cancer, according to recent research—and is also protective against free radicals. If you consistently do not go through your sleep phases at night, your body may end up producing less melatonin. This inhibits your immune system, and your resistance to many types of cancers.

Researchers from the United States and Iceland found that higher levels of melatonin in men's morning urine were associated with a decreased risk for prostate cancer, particularly advanced disease. None of the men had prostate cancer in the beginning of the study, but during the five-year follow-up, 6.4 percent were diagnosed with prostate cancer. This group also had problems falling and staying asleep. After adjusting for age, the researchers concluded that men with sleep problems were 1.6 to 2.1 times more likely to develop prostate cancer than those without sleep problems.

Lack of sleep and exposure to lights during sleep also will disrupt your production of melatonin. This is the reason that sleeping with the TV on may not be such a great idea, or any electronic device that emits light for that matter.

Excess cortisol weakens your immunity, especially white blood cells, natural killer cells, monocytes, and macrophages. Weak immune cells entice cancer cells to have a feast in your body.

Cortisol levels typically peak at dawn, after hours of sleep, and decline throughout the day. If cortisol continues to be released throughout the whole day, not just in the morning, then this is considered counterproductive and may actually contribute to cancer progression. And as I have mentioned, excess cortisol is usually released from improper stress management. For instance, poor sleep patterns are a stressor to the body and cause a release of excess cortisol.

TIPS FOR BETTER SLEEP

You need to approach sleep as you would every other aspect of your health. It is just as important as diet, exercise, supplementation, and stress reduction—everything else outlined in the CM. Give it the same attention. Here are some tips to help your sleep be more restful:

GET THE RIGHT AMOUNT

The right amount of sleep, based on much research, is seven hours. Although it's a common belief that eight hours of sleep is required for optimal health, a six-year study of more than one million adults ages

30 to 102 has shown that people who get only six to seven hours a night have a lower death rate. Individuals who sleep eight hours or more, or less than four hours a night, were shown to have a significantly higher death rate. For many patients, seven hours of sleep is a lot and it simply does not happen. Just work toward the goal of seven hours. For example, if you typically get four to five hours per night, moving up to six hours is a huge success, and makes a great impact on your overall sleep quality.

DIM THE LIGHTS AT NIGHT
Sleep in complete darkness. Start dimming the lights about three hours before bedtime. Light exposure affects the production of your night-time sleep hormone, melatonin.

GO EASY ON CAFFEINE AND ALCOHOL AT NIGHT
The half-life of caffeine is six hours, which is the time it takes your body take to get rid of one-half the amount of caffeine in your body. Some people don't have a problem sleeping after an after dinner espresso. But if any level of caffeine keeps you up, stay away from it for up to six hours before bedtime. Having a glass of red wine with dinner is also fine and may help initiate sleep. However, more than two glasses and your sleep quality suffers.

CONTROL YOUR MONKEY BRAIN BY RESTING YOUR BRAIN ON PAPER
Write down your next day's to-do list before going to sleep, which stops you from lying in the dark thinking about what needs to be done.

DISCONNECT FROM ELECTRONICS IN YOUR BEDROOM
No computers, no TV and no smartphone in your bedroom. Your bedroom is a sanctuary only for sleep and intimacy.

NO HEAVY MEALS AT NIGHT, ESPECIALLY SIMPLE, REFINED CARBS
Big meals at night make your body work too hard during sleep and interfere with sleep quality. Remember, quality sleep is just as important as quantity. That's why, if you notice when you pig out at night (and I have done so many times), you'll notice a hangover feeling, or what I call pig

out hangover. Some whole grain carbs at the right time, mainly in the evening, actually can be helpful for better sleep.

A little carbohydrate with turkey increases the levels of an amino acid called tryptophan, which helps with sleep. But the emphasis is on "little."

INVEST IN A GOOD MATTRESS

It's worth the research—time and price. While no single bed is perfect for everyone, many people swear by memory foam mattresses for a better night's rest rather than box springs. Also, you should flip your mattress every month and replace it every seven years, if not sooner, depending on wear and comfort. Although I am not tied to any particular brand, the Tempurpedic mattress has gotten high ratings in numerous consumer reports. Bottom line: find the best mattress you can afford. It's a game changer in your sleep quality.

Finally, let's be holistic, but realistic. There will be times where getting more than four or five hours of sleep is not an options. Life happens. A family crisis, flight delays, deadline with work, baby in the house or even a good party that goes on all night (and you must party). Short-term sleep deprivation will not weaken your body much. At some point soon after, you will have to make up for your sleep debt, so make sure you do.

CM Profile: David, age 54

How CM helps: How to live a better, and longer, life

With his diagnosis—no cancer, but an enlarged prostate—David knew that the odds were stacked against him and that one day he would get cancer. He wanted into increase his chances that it may not happen for 20 or maybe even 30 years.

"I wanted to do everything I could to maintain my health and keep my condition status quo," he says. He did not need to make radical changes in his life. He had faithfully taken supplements since his 30s, and was a low--carb, no sugar kind of guy. "It was more about how do I make my lifestyle better?"

Already dedicated to four to six days of exercise, David examined his diet and began to follow some of the CM guidelines like buying more organic produce and meat, cutting out white sugar, limiting drinking to a single glass of wine and one cup of coffee. "For the first time in a while, I was able to have more restful sleep," he says.

Early on, David underwent two random prostate biopsies, both revealing High Grade Prostatic Intraepithelial Neoplasm (HGPIN) – these are pre-cancer prostate cells. His PSA when we first met was 5.8ng/ml. When I saw him at the clinic back then we introduced him to the CM and he began to implement it diligently. For two years his PSA marginally decreased to a 4.7ng/ml when we decided it would be a good idea to obtain prostate tissue but this time from an targeted, more accurate biopsy. Although his PSA dropped, we wanted to make sure we were not missing something. The result of his last targeted prostate biopsy proved no HGPIN and no prostate cancer.

What he has discovered about the CM is that you do not need to make massive changes to see results. Everyone is different and everyone has different needs. "Hearing dietary and health advice from various sources can overwhelm you, and make it tough to stay focused on your needs and goals," says David. "With the CM, I was able to easily add it to my existing life, find a comfort zone, and work on the areas I need to improve."

His most recent PSA is 5.4 ng/ml, which is not significant enough to suspect prostate cancer due to his large prostate of 90grams. Larger benign prostates produce more PSA men. Today David is in excellent overall health, very active and enjoying life with his wife.

CHAPTER 7

21-DAY RESET PLAN

Commitment is an act, not a word

—Jean-Paul Sartre

WHAT EXACTLY CAUSED your prostate cancer? There is no one specific thing, but rather a multitude of causes. Yes, your genes may have played a role, but how you live, what you eat, and how your body rids environmental toxins can contribute to your current and future health.

Remember, while you may have the prostate cancer gene your environment can express those genes or keep them asleep. In other words, the cancer gene is either turned on or turned off depending on your exposure to environmental carcinogenic chemicals.

The best cancer treatment in the world won't help you in the end if you first don't clean up the cancer's home—your body. This is why, in my opinion, your cancer may return an estimated 35 percent of the time after initial treatment. It is also not uncommon for patients to first develop prostate cancer, think they are home free after treatment, and then be diagnosed later with colon, kidney, or any other type of cancer. You need to make sure your body and all its systems are cleansed and working at an optimal level if you want to heal and live longer and better. In other words, if you do not clean the biological soil, the weeds will grow wild.

So, the first step in following the CM is a 21-Day Reset Plan to jumpstart your body into the CM way of life. It is the quickest way to reboot your body, develop health habits, and overcome any food addictions. And don't fool yourself. We all have food addictions of one kind or another.

It is only for 21 days, but requires your full dedication. The rest of the CM plan will still require discipline but not as much as the Reset plan. All your health problems will not go away by the end, but after just three weeks you will feel mentally and physically amazing. I'm not kidding. You will also begin the process of creating biological soil hostile to cancer. In the process, you will have more energy and lift the mental fog that keeps you from thinking clearly. And yes, if you have a few extra pounds, they will come off, too.

The 21-Day Reset Plan may seem daunting at first, but it is fairly simple once you get the hang of it. For three weeks, you will follow a special CaPLESS eating plan and specific routines that will get you going in your new health path. The plan will also contain specific nutrients that science has shown can strengthen your natural detoxification system. This type of new eating will take planning, I know, but you want to begin feeding your body and mind only the best foods and thoughts to live your best life forward.

You may be asking, "What if I am cancer-free after treatment? Do I need to do this?" No one is 100 percent cancer-free. I am not either. We all have cancer cells harboring somewhere in our bodies, all the time. The holistic view of prostate cancer is that if there are cancer cells in your prostate, you have to assume they reside elsewhere as well. In other words, your whole body is "cancering," not just your prostate. Again, I can't tell you the amount of times I have seen prostate cancer successfully treated, only to then have the patient return with prostate cancer recurrence, or some other type. Don't be stubborn here and take your foot off the pedal and think you are completely cancer-free after treatment. You are not.

So, let's roll up our sleeves, man up, and get to work.

I have outlined the entire daily schedule of the 21-day eating plan at www.ThriveDontOnlySurvive.com. There you will find menus for daily meals and snacks, along with a timetable of when to take your supplements as part of the CM selected supplementation. You will also begin to introduce movement into your everyday life and follow the exercise programs I have designed based on your fitness level and prostate diagnosis.

Finally, during these 21 days, you also follow practices to help cleanse your body of built-up toxins and help you adopt and adjust to CM principles so they become a natural part of your new lifestyle. They are easy to do, and you will feel the effects of them almost immediately. But before you begin your 21-Day Reset, let's examine why you need to this detoxification to begin with.

CLEANING YOUR HOUSE OF TOXINS

As I previously discussed, recent science has demonstrated that environmental chemicals can influence the expression of cancer genes and turn cancer cells on and off. We are bombarded daily with a slew of environmental toxins, most with unpronounceable names, that seem to be able to penetrate our cells and make them malignant. While there have been no randomized clinical studies to conclusively prove prostate cancer is caused by environmental chemicals, there is much research that indicates a significant link.

What toxins are we talking about here? A toxin is any substance that directly causes physical harm or interferes with the normal functioning of your body. Your body makes some toxins from normal metabolism (called endotoxins), while others are found in the environment (exotoxins).

There are thousands of man-made exotoxins in our environment and in the food we eat. Why then, if toxins are practically everywhere and such a serious health risk, doesn't everyone develop cancer at some point?

It was the father of toxicology, Paracelsus, who proclaimed in the sixteenth century that, "the poison is in the dose." Even toxic substances can be safe as long as the amounts remain below a certain threshold. Yet, our modern-day problem is twofold: many of us are bombarded by an avalanche of chemicals on a daily basis and some people, for unknown reason, are better able to detoxify these chemical invaders than others. An example of this is "Uncle Bob," who smoked all his life and died at age 96. But you are not Uncle Bob, and neither am I.

Regardless, the 21-Day Reset Plan will begin the process to protect you against this chemical avalanche, and in the process begin to rebuild and renew your body. But first it is important to know about a few of these environmental toxins and, most importantly, where they are found so you can limit your exposure. The three you should be mindful about are plastics, heavy metals, and pesticides.

Let's begin with plastics.

Daily Schedule

*Follow this routine as close as possible every day during your **21-Day Reset**.*

- *Wake up between 5:00 a.m. and 6:00 a.m.*

- *Do your bathroom routine complete with brushing and hydrotherapy*

- *Drink an 8-oz glass of purified water*

- *Sit quietly for 5 to 10 minutes and take five deep breaths*

- *Give thanks for what you have. You can express this in low voice, in your head or in prayer*

- *Exercise for 30 minutes (get it done before your day begins. You will feel charged for the day and won't be tempted to make excuses and blow it off.)*

- *After exercising, brush your dry skin then get in the shower*

- *Take a shower and finish with 5 to 10 minutes of hot/cold contrast, always end with cold*

- *Details on www.ThriveDontOnlySurvive.com*

PLASTICS

The surge of plastics as a commodity was highlight in the 1967 film, "The Graduate." There is a classic scene where Benjamin Braddock (played by

Dustin Hoffman), a recent college graduate with no well-defined aim in life, is pulled aside by businessman Mr. McGuire.

> Mr. McGuire: I just want to say one word to you. Just one word.
> Benjamin: Yes, sir.
> Mr. McGuire: Are you listening? Benjamin: Yes, I am.
> Mr. McGuire: Plastics.
> Benjamin: Exactly how do you mean?
> Mr. McGuire: There's a great future in plastics. Think about it. Will you think about it?

Indeed, Mr. McGuire was right. Plastics are everywhere—from water bottles to Tupperware—which means the chemicals that make them up are everywhere, too. There are quite a number of chemical in plastics, and two in particular that cause problems: bisphenol A (BPA) and phthalates.

BPA and phthalates are found in plastics and BPA is also especially found on the inner lining of canned foods like tomato sauce, vegetables, and soups, where it helps avoid corrosion of the metal.

BPA enters the body through the liquid or food we consume. For instance, it can leach into the water when a plastic bottle is heated or exposed to prolonged sunlight or stress. BPA naturally leaches into food from cans within time. Once in our body, BPA and phthalates can disrupt the normal functioning of hormones, like testosterone and estrogen, which can make cancer cells more active.

In fact, one study showed that even very low concentrations of BPA initiated the proliferation of cancer cells.

I am not sharing this information to alarm you and have you think all those bottles of water you drank is the cause of your prostate cancer. It may not be. And prostate cancer is not that simple. Besides, BPA and phthalates are ubiquitous and unavoidable. What you can do is lower your exposure and provide key nutrients that will help you detoxify from exposure.

LOWER YOUR EXPOSURE

Avoiding plastic bottles is the easiest way to protect yourself from BPA. But if you do use them, choose wisely. Plastic bottles have a recycling code at the bottom of the bottle that looks like a triangular arrow around a number. Avoid these numbers: 3, 6, and 7, as they contain the highest amounts of BPA. Plastics with number 1, 2, 4, and 5 are safer plastics and contain the lowest levels of BPA and phthalates. Also, avoid or at least reduce your intake of canned foods. Instead, opt for frozen choices or the whole foods.

Other tips: Use glass containers instead of plastic to store your food. Also, avoid purchasing either canned salmon or canned sardines in vinyl-lined cans, which may contain BPA. I recommend contacting the manufacturers of these products to find out which are using BPA-free cans. If you cannot find BPA-free choices, you may want to consider purchasing the fish in another (noncanned) form. Vital Choice (www.vitalchoice.com) offers an excellent assortment of wild BPA-free fish and sardines.

HEAVY METALS

Another group of environmental toxins worth mentioning are heavy metals, especially cadmium. Cadmium is a known carcinogen and is linked to prostate cancer in several preliminary studies. Other research has found an increased concentration of cadmium in prostates with cancer when compared to normal glands. And a 2013 study found a link between dietary cadmium and hormone cancers like prostate, breast, and ovarian, especially in Western countries.

Lower Your Exposure: Food and cigarette smoke are the largest sources of cadmium exposure in the general population. Smokers have a daily cadmium intake that may be twice that of nonsmokers. Occupational exposures may also occur among welders, metal workers, or those who make cadmium products, such as batteries or plastics. You can further protect yourself by making sure you get adequate amounts of calcium, iron, and zinc—which you can do by following CaPLESS eating—as the absorption of cadmium is increased when you are deficient in these nutrients. Taking your selenium supplements from high selenized yeast, SelenoExcell, NAC, and modified citrus pectin as part of the CM's Smart Supplementation also can help eliminate cadmium in the body.

PESTICIDES
There appears to be a correlation between pesticide exposure and prostate cancer. For example, many occupational studies show an increased incidence of prostate cancer incidence and/or mortality among farmers and pesticide applicators. One in vitro study of human prostate cancer cells showed that several types of pesticides like organochlorine pesticides and fungicides, caused proliferation of prostate cancer cells.

Lower Your Exposure: The best way to avoid pesticides is to eat organic foods whenever possible. CaPLESS eating advocates organic choices for 4 and 5 foods, which are the foundation of your 21-day eating plan as well as common fruits and vegetables on the Environmental Working Group's "dirty dozen" list, which highlights food with the highest exposure to pesticides.

HOW DETOXIFICATION WORKS
Your body already possesses the best detoxification system. Your digestive/elimination system does an impressive job keeping unwanted junk out of your system when you eat and move it quickly out of your body. Even if harmful substances make it through your digestion and into your bloodstream, the liver is there to detect it, break it down, and help to eliminate it. Your skin helps to protect your body from toxin absorption and excretes toxins through sweat. Your lungs feed your cells rich

oxygen with every deep breath and also strengthen your lymphatic system, which moves waste and toxins out of the body.

While it all sounds simple, your internal detoxification system is actually quite complex and involves various enzymes and chemical reactions to convert toxins to nontoxic substances so your body can more easily move them out.

What you need to keep in mind is that right now you are at the height of your toxin exposure and your detox system is operating at its weakest level. The 21-Day Reset is designed to reverse that.

DAILY HABITS AND RITUALS

Every day during the next three weeks you will adopt various lifestyle habits and rituals. They are designed to help you detoxify the main organs of your body's detoxification system: skin, liver, elimination, and lungs. This is done through steady eating of specific 4s and 5s foods, daily exercise, and hygiene practices. They don't take much effort, but you will be amazed at how effective they work and how they can change how you feel. I am confident that you will probably want to continue them even after the 21-Day Reset has finished as yet another means live your best life going forward.

SKIN (BRUSHING, SWEATING, AND HYDROTHERAPY)
Besides being your largest organ, your skin is your first protection against toxins and chemicals. Many toxins are released through your sweat and skin, and brushing helps rid toxins from your skin and prevent them from going back into your system. Follow this brushing routine:

- Dry brush your entire body (except your face) for three minutes before bathing, gently but thoroughly, three times a week
- The recommended approach is right before showering
- Use a loofah sponge, dry brush, or dry towel
- Brush in one-stroke movements. Do not brush too hard—your skin should not redden too much.

- Brush from the outermost part of your body (hands and feet) toward your abdomen and chest.
- Try to reach as many areas of your body you can.

After brushing, take a regular shower and end it with a series of hot and cold water contrasts known as hydrotherapy. This jump-starts your circulation and increases the production of glutathione (GSH), an antioxidant that protects cells from free radicals and inflammation. First, make the water as hot as you can tolerate without scalding yourself and let it pour over your entire body for three minutes. Then turn the water to cold (as cold as you can tolerate) for 30 seconds. One hot/cold contrast equals one cycle. Do three cycles every morning and

always finish with cold to stimulate all your systems and contain core body heat.

Finally, switch your antiperspirant for an herbal or natural ingredient deodorant. You do not want to inhibit sweating, as it's a natural process and an important avenue of body detoxification.

LIVER AND DETOXIFICATION

Virtually all chemical toxins, environmental and the ones your body creates, are fat-soluble, which means they dissolve only in fatty or oily solutions and not in water.

This is where your liver comes into play. It works hard to covert fat-soluble substances to water soluble ones so they then can be more easily eliminated. You can help your liver by eliminating substances that are especially burdensome to its function, such as alcohol and caffeine, and preservatives and dyes found in processed foods. And as part of the 21-Day Reset diet plan you will consume foods that specifically help to nourish and strengthen the liver, such as beets, artichokes, and their fresh juices. Botanical herbs and nutrients also help liver function and improve detoxification. These include: milk thistle, NAC, and schisandra berry extract.

COLON HEALTH AND ELIMINATION

For detoxification to be successful, you need to move out the toxins and chemicals from your body. Your elimination system—colon function and bowel movement—is the final stage of detoxification. You need to keep your colon healthy to encourage regular and thorough elimination.

Many 4s and 5s foods you will consume, such as raw vegetables, fruits, and cooked grains like brown rice, oats, barley, millet, and quinoa, contain high amounts of fiber to help soften stools, promote regular bowel movement, and keep your gut clean and running smoothly. Adopting regular exercise, especially aerobic exercise, as outlined in Chapter 4, "CaPLESS Movement," also can help promote positive bowel function.

LUNGS (DEEP BREATHING)

Practice relaxed deep breathing twice a day for 10 minutes—in the morning before you begin your day and at night before bedtime. This kind of breathing exercise calms your sympathetic (fight or flight) nervous system, which will help you manage your stress. It also increases oxygen delivery to your cells, which cancer cells hate as they thrive in oxygen-free environments. It also promotes circulation of your lymphatic system and work as the sewage system of your body to take out the junk.

- Find a quiet and comfortable place free from distractions
- Sit straight with your belly and chest relaxed
- Take a deep breath, inhaling to a four count then holding for a four count and slowly exhaling to a four count
- Inhale through your nose and expand your belly outward (not your chest)
- Repeat up to 10 times

TO DO During Your 21-Day Reset

• *Sleep a minimum of seven hours a night*

• *Wake up at 5:00–6:00 a.m. and go to bed by 10:00 p.m.*

• *Begin regular exercise with a balance of strength training, aerobics, and stretching. (Visit www.ThriveDontOnlySurvive.com)for sample workout programs based on your current fitness level on prostate cancer diagnosis.)*

• *Spend 20 minutes a day in mediation or silence. It breaks up your busy day and gives your body and mind a time to rest and renew.*

DON'TS During Your 21-Day Reset

• *Eliminate caffeine (coffee, tea, etc.) I know your morning coffee or afternoon tea may see harsh, and while these beverages offer many health benefits, you want to break away from any type of addictive foods for the next three weeks.*

• *Avoid all processed foods. If it comes in a box or a package, you don't want it. They are full of chemicals and additives, which can increase your body's toxic load.*

• *Avoid nighttime snacking as it may interfere with restorative sleep.*

• *If you experience hunger pangs, drink a full glass of water. Nighttime hunger will diminish with time.*

GETTING STARTED ON YOUR 21-DAY RESET PLAN

Discipline is the cornerstone of the CM. Like any other aspect of life, from work to relationships, you need discipline to reach your maximum potential. The next 21 days will require planning, commitment, and discipline. But the good news is that I've outlined the planning for you. I've created a daily schedule for you to follow each week, so you know what to do, when, and most importantly why. It is up to you to stick to it, but I also offer tips and advice to help you through any rough patches to make sure to make it through the entire 21 days. Here's what you can expect for each week.

Week One

This is will be the most challenging week by far. Everything is new and different. But in many ways it is also the most important. This is when you get kicked out of your comfort zone and your old ways of doing things.

Change can be tough and expect to feel some level of discomfort until you begin to get comfortable with your new habits. Hang in there. Trust me: by the end of the week you feel lighter with a clearer mind, and more natural energy—you won't even miss your coffee!

You will also get use to feeling full and satisfied with less food. There is an old saying, "The less you eat, the longer you live." There is a lot of truth to that. By only eating 4s and 5s during the next 21 days you will notice how you can feel better by eating smarter meals, and you will be surprised to learn to will not feel the urge to satisfy hunger pangs with crappy food filled with tons of sugar, simple carbs, and caffeine. Stick with it and it will get easier.

Week Two

You are going to feel really good. The new habits don't feel so new any-more and get easier, and the positive physical benefits will significantly increase. You may even have lost a few pounds and notice an overall improvement in your quality of life. You are cruising.

Week Three

By week three the program has becomes old hat. By now your body has flushed out much of the toxins and waste from your body and mind feels the clearest it has been in a long time. Your outlook in life is more posi-tive. Your skin has become smoother and cleaner, and because you have reduced levels of inflammatory chemicals your immune system is now stronger and your body has created the hostile environment to begin fighting cancer cells.

CM Profile: Richard, 47

How CM helped: Control his stress and recognize his health beyond prostate

After his prostate surgery, Richard was able to lose weight and get fit with CM, but he still battled his greatest health obstacle: stress. He ran a successful small business, but for years had let constant worrying dictate his life. He found the CM approach to stress reduction and management was able to break that cycle and provide much-needed balance to his new lifestyle.

"I knew there was no magic bullet, but CM showed me how to make the small changes and embrace new techniques to keep my stress under control," he says. "I used to wake up in the night worried about life and my health, but now I am more restful and the episodes of hives I faced on a regular basis are now gone."

Richard adopted a regular yoga program and followed a daily mindfulness practice that included breathing exercises. Being more in tune with his body and mind, and recognizing how each influenced the other, showed him how situations and actions affected his well-being. "I changed my mind-set about what was important and not to take everything so serious," he says. "Now when I feel myself becoming stressed, I can throw an internal switch and center myself. I have learned that some things can wait for the next day, and I no longer let my sleep get disrupted by negative thoughts."

A clearer mind also has opened his mind to other aspects of his life. "My new approach to living goes beyond my prostate cancer. I know I have to live better overall, which can protect me from other health risks, too."

Details of Richard's CaP history: I met Richard, now 51 years-old, three years ago after his prostatectomy for a after cancer wellness visit. At the time he was 191 pounds at 5 ' 11 height. His prostate pathology report was staged at T2c, Gleason 7 with negative margins. Richard had a strong paternal and maternal family history of cancer. As a father of two teenagers and a successful businessman, he was eager to start the CaPLESS method. His recent clinical visit was impressive: undetectable PSA, he lost 25 pounds, lost 3 inches from his waist and all cardiovascular blood markers at optimal levels. Richard is an example of making prostate cancer an opportunity to live your best life forward.

CHAPTER 8

BRINGING IT ALL HOME

We are what we repeatedly do. Excellence, then,
is not an act, but a habit.

—ARISTOTLE

NOW THAT YOU hopefully have a full understanding of the CaPLESS Method and how it works, you are probably saying to yourself, "Whoa! Dr. Geo, how the heck am I supposed to do all this?"

Relax man. Take a deep breath. As Bob Marley once said, "Everything will be all right."

Understand and apply the key principles: Eat optimally, move often, sleep well, quiet your mind, and consume selected supplements. Figure out where you are most deficient and focus there. The CaPLESS Method is a journey, not a destination. You do not have to be perfect, but you do have to improve continuously. It will all come together with effort and time. There are three elements to success with the CM: Persistence, Commitment, and Discipline.

COMMITMENT

I will be blunt: You need to be 100 percent in. Not 50 percent, 75 percent, or even 90 percent. It is all or nothing. Prostate cancer is your wake up call. Don't squander this opportunity to live your absolute best life. I am not asking you to be perfect, but I am asking you to be 100 percent committed to living your best life and moving forward. You deserve it. And so does your family.

PERSISTENCE

There are times when living the CM will be a challenge. No doubt about it. Parties, travel, everyday events all make it tough to stick to a structured lifestyle plan like the CM. But don't worry. The CM is designed to take those dips and valleys into consideration. A night out with the boys? Yep, that can also be a doozy. No worries, between this book and other available resources I'll make available to you, you'll be able to join all of life's fun events while staying the course. Plus, I never said you can't your cake, and eat it too.

DISCIPLINE

This is the most important trait to be successful with the CM for life. Self-discipline is a learned behavior. It requires every day practice and repetition.

This type of thought pattern is part of the process, but gets easier with practice and time. Within four to six weeks, you will notice how your food choices, exercise regimen, and supplement intakes will feel more automatic and a natural part of your life. You will not have to think about what to do next all the time. The CM becomes a way of life, which is the ultimate goal.

The self-discipline needed for the CM carries over into other aspects of your life, too. According to a 2013 study by Wilhelm Hoffman, people with high self-control are happier than those without. The study discovered this is true because the self-disciplined subjects were more capable of dealing with goal conflicts. These people spent less time debating whether to indulge in behaviors detrimental to their health, and were able to make positive decisions more easily.

The self-disciplined did not allow their choices to be dictated by impulses or feelings. Instead, they made informed, rational decisions on a daily basis without feeling overly stressed or upset.

Here's the deal—improving your self-discipline means changing your normal routine, which is usually uncomfortable and awkward at first. But hang in there. Within three to six weeks you will be on autopilot. While you will likely intelligently deviate from the program at times (and I even suggest you do so), you will revert back to who you are now: a CaPLESS thriver.

Think about this for a second: has any worthwhile venture in your life come easy to you? Ever? Aren't you successful in some area of life? Was it always easy? Or did you have to work your butt off to make it happen? It is the same with the CaPLESS Method. Similar elements to success are required here.

At first, frustration and confusion may set in. (Is chicken a 3 or a 2 on the Food Rating System? Geez, I'd like to eat a little piece of cake at my buddy's party tonight, but I don't want to make my cancer worse.)

Also, you know that there are no solid "don'ts" in this program. I will never tell you not to eat anything. You will never hear from me to eat low-fat this, low-calorie that, or load up on protein.

HOW TO TALK TO YOUR DOCTOR ABOUT THE CM?

You are never alone while following the CM. Your family is involved of course, but what about others? What about your doctor?

The truth is, your physician likely has little or no interest in speaking with you about the CM, natural medicine or any nontraditional approach to prostate cancer. In fact, if you bring it up, he may say one of three things:

1. There's no proof any of that stuff works.
2. That's quackery. Don't waste your time or money on it.
3. I don't know much about this approach to lifestyle and nutrition to comment on it.

My suggestion: If your physician's answer is 1 or 2, consider finding a more open-minded doctor. The reality is that there are deficiencies in both forms of medicine: the conventional and the natural, and each form, when used properly, fulfills the deficiency of the other.

There are many physicians, particularly urologists, who will not look at you like you have three heads when you tell them you are interested in following the CM program.

If you are at a point where you are seeing an oncologist, then you will have a tougher time having them accept your decision to follow the CM. Oncologists typically don't mind "diet and exercise" but cringe at the use of supplements since dietary supplements are so poorly understood by conventional wisdom.

Bottom line: You are the captain of your ship, so work with a physician who will respect your position in being a proactive about your health. No one doctor alone can cure you. You have to cure yourself.

Don't take this the wrong way and be anti-medicine. I am not disparaging medical doctors. I have had the privilege of working with progressive medical doctors and urologists in multidisciplinary settings for most of my career.

However, I have seen firsthand the power of an integrative practice where treatments are followed with peri-operative holistic care. The outcomes have been outstanding. But I also know Western physicians who are critical of an integrative approach and discourage patient to pursue this path by hiding behind the no evidence excuse.

One can only find what they look for. There is a plethora of evidence suggesting the different elements of the CaPLESS Method work. But only if you look for such evidence.

WHAT TO DO WHEN YOU TRAVEL?

The CM is a lifestyle, which means you follow it throughout all aspects of your life, even when you are away from your usual routine and environment.

This means that when the flight attendant asks if you would like peanuts, cookies, or pretzels or soft drinks, you say, "No, thank you."

Remember you are always in control with the CM, and one of its best features is that you can always take it with you. For example, here's how you can pack along the CM when you travel:

1. Eat a quality meal before leaving for the airport. It can be a five-minute smoothie or leftover meal from the night before. No time to make something? Eat an apple and a palm full of mixed nuts.
2. Find a health food market near the hotel. Stock up on fruits, health snacks, and quality water. If your room has an oven and you plan to cook, then stock up on anything you plan to cook.
3. Don't forget your workout gear. Bring your TRX, resistance bands, and any other easy-to-store exercise equipment if you'd like. Body weight exercises work fine too. Twenty minutes a day is all that's required, but make each minute count.
4. Sleep as much as you can.
5. Have fun. If you are traveling for vacation or business, there are always opportunities to have fun. Go for walks around town. Check out a local yoga studio.
6. Don't overdrink. A cocktail or two is OK, but more than that becomes messy. Your sleep quality takes a hit, and it is simply anti-CaPLESS.

THE ECONOMICS OF THE CM

Your new, healthier lifestyle is an investment in your life. And any good investment involves some initial upstart funding.

Here's the deal: We have been conditioned to think that we can only pay premium dollars for material items like cars, vacations, houses, etc. There is less value on spending hard-earned money on living your best.

You need to change your thinking of how you spend your money. Buying more foods that you usually don't eat in high amounts, like fruits, vegetables, nuts, and seeds, can increase your food bill up to an extra $1.50 per day. If you go organic (and you should as much as possible; see sidebar, "Go Organic"), the cost can rise anywhere from $1 to $2 more per food item than conventional produce. We are talking an additional $240 a year for one person who is eating more organic fruits and vegetables. If the whole family is involved, then multiply $240 times the number of family members.

Why is eating healthier so expensive? Our government is out to lunch.

Policymakers do not offer subsidies or financial support for growing and buying vegetables and fruits. Current farm subsidies are geared toward refined grain products like corn syrup and sugar—which make up most of the foods in the 1 and 2 on the Food Rating System that contribute the most to cancer and disease. Do you wonder why healthcare cost is so high? I won't get on my political rant, but you know what I mean.

Here's what you should do not to be sticker shocked by your new grocery habits:

Create a health budget for you and your family, and stick to it like you would any other serious budget, like your business or household expenses. Your health budget includes the cost of your new food; exercise equipment; clothing; and gym memberships, dietary supplements, and other health activities like retreats.

Be as diligent with your health budget as you are about your mortgage and car bills. In other words, once you have your health budget in place, then other discretionary expenses come after that, so in case you run out of cash, your and your family's health don't take a hit.

A FINAL WORD

I feel privileged to be part of your wellness/anticancer journey. I really trust you will take the bull by the horns and apply the principles of the CaPLESS Method. If you (or a partner) are reading this, you have an opportunity to create a strong, energetic, longer life. There's no BS here. Only real results when this program is applied diligently.

For some of you, this lifestyle program has validated much of what you already knew, to some degree. You may just need a little tweaking here and there. Just don't intellectualize the CaPLESS Method without taking action.

Don't say, "It's common sense, I know what to do," and then do nothing. I have seen this happen. This is not a diet or just a gimmicky workout regimen. This is a systematic, evidence-based lifestyle intervention that has been validated by science and thousands of patients I have seen.

Bottom line: The CM works, and it works well in keeping your body strong and cancer under control when diligently applied. Also, this program will not change much with the times. I have tried to put together specific lifestyle principles that are timeless. And remember, once you learn and apply these guidelines, you can always break them intelligently—guilt-free.

Don't be surprised if it takes a little while for this lifestyle to become automatic. Be patient, enjoy the process, and if you fall off, then quickly get "back on the horse." And if you go off the program for several days, do another 21-Day Reset to get your mind right and your body back on track.

Now it is up to you to make it real. This book is filled with only words unless you are fully committed to a stronger you. This is your time to renew, rebuild, and reclaim your health. Stay in touch, and let me know how it goes for you at www.ThriveDontOnlySurvive.com.

Learn from other CaPLESS thrivers who continue to broadcast how they are challenged with the program and how they are kicking butt. If you are committed to you living your best life despite your diagnosis, then I am committed to helping you. Have an amazing rest of your life.

Thrive—don't only survive!

Go Organic

Eating organic foods when possible is important for the CaPLESS Method. Organic foods simply have less crap that promotes disease and cancer. Since organic foods raise your food cost, mainly eat these foods organically if you have to choose:

- *apples*

- *peaches*

- *sweet bell peppers*

- *celery*

- *nectarines*

- *strawberries*

- *cherries*

- *pears*

- *grapes (imported)*

- *spinach*

- *lettuce*

- *potatoes*

ACKNOWLEDGMENTS

WHEN I FIRST began writing this book about five years ago (I'm embarrassed to admit it took that long), I thought it depended all on me: my ability to write, be creative, research, design a nice cover, come up with an attractive title, etc.

Reality soon set in, and I realized there is a crew of people who helped make this book happen.

Thank you:

My editor, Matthew Solan, who kept pressing until this potentially complex material became user friendly to you, the reader.

My real teachers—my patients, who trust me as an integral part of their medical team to guide them in rebuilding their bodies and transition in becoming CaPLESS thrivers. Thank you for the privilege to fulfill my passion and to be of service in your journey toward health and healing.

My students who have trusted me in sharing my clinical experiences. I hope you learn as much from me as I learn from you.

The dream team at NYU Urology: Huang, Stifelman Nitti, Alukal, Borin, Brucker, Rosenblum, Smilen, Balar, Shapiro, Zhao, Makarov, Loeb, and Telegrafi. Thank you for trusting me with your patients even without yet understanding how acupuncture, naturopathic, or functional medicine works. It's OK. I, too, am still exploring how it works.

Dr. Taneja, whose unwavering focus on academic excellence is so inspiring and contagious. Thank you for referrals of your prostate cancer patients who trust in me when they come from you.

The boss, Dr. Herbert Lepor—thank you for being an amazing chairman, distinguished surgeon, and outstanding role model for me and the rest of us at our department. Most of all, thank you for taking a chance on me and allowing me to develop an integrative and functional urology segment of our department—a concept that is gaining ground but still foreign in many conventional settings. I am forever grateful for the opportunity and privilege to work alongside the greats at NYU Urology.

Erica Nelom—my assistant and the one who keeps me organized at the clinic. Thank you for your tireless work in helping our fabulous patients see me. I would never be able to do what I do without you.

Dr. Robert Valenzuela—my friend and excellent urologist. It's been more than 12 years since you introduced me to the wonderful specialty of urology. I cannot thank you enough.

Dr. Aaron Katz—the first holistic urologist and my mentor for so many years. My life changed when you gave me an opportunity to work with you at the Holistic Urology Center at Columbia. My family and I thank you so much.

Dr. Eugene Zamperion—my first naturopathic urology professor and friend. Thank you for teaching me how to see urology patients holistically and not just from the waist down. Much respect, mon.

Naturopathic oncologists—Drs. Lise Alschuler, Daniel Rubin, and Tina Kaczor. I have learned tons from you and am so happy you chose oncology as your specialty, from which I have benefited so much.

Dr. Peter D'Adamo—naturopathic doctor and a great friend. You were the first to teach me what success looks like as an ND with your *New York Times* best-selling book, *Eat Right for Your Blood Type*, and simply by the one-on-one side talks that were so instrumental before going to naturopathic school. I remain forever grateful to you and Martha for taking a chance and hiring me and NAP.

You, too, Martha D'Adamo. Your graceful leadership while running North American Pharmacal and raising your two beautiful girls is something Johanna and I still admire. The memories at NAP, working alongside the Tuz, are ones I will always cherish. Thank you for the opportunity to work for you.

My integrative and functional medicine colleagues, Drs. Joel Evans, Frank Lipman, Ronald Hoffman, and Aviva Romm and many others who I simply can't mention as I run out of space. You know who you are. Thank you for your referrals and your friendship.

My good friend and partner David Guinther for being an example of a CaPLESS thriver—not only a survivor—and for sharing your passion with me in helping others battling prostate cancer become thrivers with quality nutrition. Your friendship and partnership at XYwellness is one I am extremely grateful for.

My brothers, Micheal and Luis, for always being there for me throughout my life and always showing me brotherly love.

My sisters, Maria and Rosalba, although you live far, I always feel your love and support.

Ernestina, my mom, who raised us with the "iron fist"—I thank you for that. I am not sure the outcome of my life would have been so good any other way growing up in the tough streets of the Bronx. Te quiero mucho, mami.

To my extended family and friends, way too many to mention, but you know who you are. The support, especially during those hard times, is one that is deeply felt in my heart forever. You have no idea how much you have to do with the completion of this book.

To the light of my eyes, my three beautiful kids, Mia, Gianna, and Leonardo. You three give me the energy and purpose I need to work hard. Words cannot describe how much I love you. Thank you for under-standing when daddy is out late at night writing at a coffee shop.

And finally, to my rock and the best life-partner anyone could ever have, my wife, Johanna. I am grateful beyond measure to have you in my life. You have been so incredibly patient and understanding with me throughout this journey. Thank you for being you. I love you.

INDEX

stress product, 28, 79

costs of CaPLESS Method, 106–107

COX-2 enzyme, 57, 64

crapless eating, 38–41, 100

cruciferous vegetables, 42–43

cryotherapy, 19

cumin, 47

curcumin (turmeric), 57, 64

curry, 47

cyberknife, 18

cyclooxygenase (COX), 53, 64

cytochrome P450 (cP450), 54

D

D'Adamo, Martha, 113

D'Adamo, Peter, 113

daily supplementation. *See* supplementation

death from prostate cancer

    exercise and, 69, 70–71

    fish consumption and, 45

    percentage of, xiv

    sitting and, 75

    something else will get you, xiv, 4–5

deciding on treatment, 19, 117

Decipher® (GenomeDx), 10, 11

deodorant over antiperspirant, 97

Designs for Health, 118

detoxification

    body's natural detox, 95–96

    colon health, 98

    daily rituals, 96–97

    environmental toxins, 91–95

    importance of, 91–92

grains, whole, 45, 87, 98

grape seed extract (GSE), 58, 64

grapes (imported), 109

green tea extract, 57–58, 64

grouper, 45

guilt indigestible, 38, 41

Guinther, David, 113

H

hazelnuts, 46

health budget, 107

heart rate monitor for exercise, 73–74

heartburn, 47

heavy metal detoxification, 58, 94–95

herbicides as carcinogens, 43, 95

herbs and spices principle, 46–47

HGPIN (high grade prostatic intraepithelial neoplasm), 9, 88

high intensity frequency ultrasound (HIFU), 19

high selenized yeast, 51, 58–59, 95

Hoffman, Dustin, 92–93

Hoffman, Ronald, 113

Hoffman, Wilhelm, 103

Holistic Urology Center (Columbia University Medical Center), xi, xv, 112

holy basil, 64

hormone depletion therapy, 77

hu zhang, 64

Huang at NYU Urology, 111

humor to de-stress, 82

hunger pangs and water, 99

husbands. *See* life partners

hydrotherapy, 92, 97

hypothalamus and word emotions, xvi

hypoxemia from sleep apnea, 84

Integrative and Functional Urology Center (NYU Langone Medical Center), xv, 115
integrative and nutritionally oriented practitioners, 119
integrative medicine
    integrative urology, 112, 113, 115
    outcomes of, 22, 105
    resources for, 117, 119
Integrative Therapeutics, 118
interleukins (IL-6), 53
iron, 95

J
Johns Hopkins, 14, 63

K
Kaczor, Tina, 112
kalc, 43
Katz, Aaron, 112
kidney stones, 43, 46
king mackerel, 45

L
laughter to de-stress, 82
Lee, Bruce, 83
Lepor, Herbert, 112
lettuce, 109
Life Extension Foundation, 117
life partners
    CaPLESS benefits, xviii, 20, 25, 41
    CaPLESS Method support, 32, 41, 54, 69
    CaPLESS Wellness retreats, 20, 28–29
    doctor visits with, 13
    exercise partners, 69

ABOUT THE AUTHOR

GEO ESPINOSA, ND, LAc, is a renowned naturopathic doctor recognized as an authority in integrative and functional urology. He has published in numerous peer-reviewed scientific journals related to integrative management of prostate conditions and urological disorders. Dr. Geo has been a medical contributor to *Men's Journal* magazine, WebMD, and major medical textbooks. He is the founder and director of the Integrative and Functional Urology Center at New York University Langone Medical Center (NYULMC) and lectures internationally on the clinical application of integrative and functional medicine in urology. Dr. Geo has been recognized as one of the top 10 Health Makers for Men's Health by sharecare.com, created by Dr. Mehmet Oz and WebMD. On his time off from work, he enjoys writing on his popular blog, DrGeo. com, and participating in outdoor activities with his wife and three kids. Dr. Geo was born to Cuban parents in the Bronx, New York, and lives in the Riverdale section of the Bronx with his family.

Matthew Solan is an award-winning health and fitness writer whose articles have appeared in *Men's Health, Men's Fitness, Muscle & Fitness, Yoga Journal,* and *Runner's World.* www.matthewsolan.com.

CAPLESS RESOURCES

Taking the CaPLESS Method to the next level
If the concepts highlighted in this book has inspired you to go all in and take your health to the next level here are some resources:

This books website: www.ThriveDontOnlySurvive.com - For handouts, tools, information and a thriving prostate cancer community

CaPLESS Retreat: www.CaPLESSretreat.com - This is an all out, full-immersion event detailing all the concepts of the CaPLESS method.

Other Useful Websites:

Dr. Geo's Blog: www.DrGeo.com - where we inspire, motivate and educate men (and women about men) on functional and integrative approaches to optimal health.

Life Extension Foundation: www.LifeExtensionFoundation.com - for science-based methods to anti-aging

NYU Smilow Comprehensive Prostate Cancer Center:
http://nyulangone.org/locations/smilow-comprehensive-prostate-cancer-center - Clinic on multidisciplinary approach towards prostate cancer

Dr. Ralph Moss' website: www.CancerDecisions.com - Provides reports on worldwide, unbiased information on cancer treatments

FOOD
To find a Farmer's Market near you www.localharvest.org

Information on Grass-fed, Organic Meats
www.eatwild.com

Environmental Working Group - Dirty Dozen food list and other environmental health information
www.ewg.org

Great resource for quality fish
Vital Choice Wild Seafood & Organics
PO Box 4121
Bellingham, WA 98227
www.vitalchoice.com

EXCELLENT PRACTITIONER DIETARY SUPPLEMENT SOURCES
XY Wellness, LLC
CaP specific nutrition
Madison, Wisconsin
www.XYwellness.com
(The author is co-founder and formulator)

Designs for Health
980 South St, Suffield, CT 06078
www.designsforhealth.com

Integrative Therapeutics
Prothrivers line
825 Challenger Drive
Green Bay, WI 54311
www.integrativepro.com

Douglas Labs
600 Boyce Road
Pittsburgh, PA 15205
www.douglaslabs.com

Pure Encapsulations
490 Boston Post Rd,
Sudbury, MA 01776
www.pureencapsulations.com

American Biosciences
Makers Ave Ultra
560 Bradley Hill Rd # 4
Blauvelt, NY 10913
www.americanbiosciences.com

New Chapter
90 Technology Drive
Brattleboro, VT 05301
www.newchapter.com

INTEGRATIVE AND NUTRITIONALLY ORIENTED PRACTITIONERS

American Association of Naturopathic Physicians (AANP) - www. Naturopathic.org
The Institute of Functional Medicine - www.functionalmedicine.org
Oncology Association of Naturopathic Physicians - www.oncanp.org

NOTES

CHAPTER 1:

Andriole GL, Crawford ED, Grubb RL 3rd, Buys SS, Chia D, Church TR, et al., PLCO Project Team. Prostate cancer screening in the randomized Prostate, Lung, Colorectal, and Ovarian Cancer Screening Trial: mortality results after 13 years of follow-up. J Natl Cancer Inst. 2012; 104:125–32.

Steinberg DM; Sauvageot J; Piantadosi S; Epstein JI Correlation Of Prostate Needle Biopsy And Radical Prostatectomy Gleason Grade In Academic And Community Settings. Am J Surg Pathol 1997;21(5):566–76.

Schröder FH, Hugosson J, Roobol MJ, Tammela TL, Ciatto S, Nelen V, et al., ERSPC Investigators. Screening and prostate-cancer mortality in a randomized European study. N Engl J Med. 2009; 360:1320–8.

NYT article Dr. Ablin
http://www.google.com/url?sa=t&rct=j&q=&esrc=s&source=web&cd=1&ved=0CCkQFjAA&url=http%3A%2F%2Fwww.nytimes.com%2F2010%2F03%2F10%2Fopinion%2F10Ablin.html&ei=pFs7UqlxuK_gA_rKgNAJ&usg=AFQjCNFpzONQUzgSZJJPdbCpWCeP_S7yBA&bvm=bv.52288139, d.dmg.

Carter HB, Pearson JD, Metter EJ, et al. Longitudinal evaluation of prostate-specific antigen levels in men with and without prostate disease. JAMA. 1992; 267: 2215–2220.

Punglia RS, Cullen J, Mcleod DG, Chen Y, D'Amico AV. Prostate-specific antigen velocity and the detection of Gleason score 7 to 10 prostate cancer. Cancer 2007; 110(9):1973–1978.

Llorente MD, Burke M, Gregory GR, et al. Prostate cancer: a significant risk factor for late-life suicide. Am J Geriatr Psychiatry. 2005; 13: 195–201.

Bayraktar Z[1], Inan EH, Bayraktar V. Effect of constipation on serum total prostate-specific antigen levels in men. Int J Urol. 2012 Jan;19(1):54-9.

D'Amico AV, Chen MH, Roehl KA, Catalona WJ. Preoperative PSA velocity and the risk of death from prostate cancer after radical prostatectomy. N Engl J Med 2004; 351(2):125–135.

Klotz L, Teahan S. Current role of PSA kinetics in the management of patients with prostate cancer. Eur Urol 2006; 5(6):471–536.

Vickers AJ, Till C, Tangen CM, Lilja H, Thompson IM. An empirical evaluation of guidelines on prostate specific antigen velocity in prostate cancer detection. J Natl Cancer Inst 2011; 103(6):462–469.

Loeb S, Sutherland DE, D'Amico AV, Roehl KA, Catalona WJ. PSA velocity is associated with Gleason score in radical prostatectomy specimen: Marker for prostate cancer aggressiveness. Urology 2008; 72(5): 1116–1120, discussion 1120.

Vlaeminck-Guillem V, Ruffion A, Andre J (May 2008). "[Value of urinary PCA3 test prostate cancer diagnosis]." *Prog. Urol.* (in French) 18 (5): 259–65.

Vickers AJ, Till C, Tangen CM, Lilja H, Thompson IM. An empirical evaluation of guidelines on prostate-specific antigen velocity in prostate cancer detection. J Natl Cancer Inst. 2011 Mar 16; 103(6): 462–9.

Lepor H[1], Llukani E[2], Sperling D[3], Fütterer JJ[4].Complications, Recovery, and Early Functional Outcomes and Oncologic Control Following

In-bore Focal Laser Ablation of Prostate Cancer. Eur Urol. 2015 May 12. pii: S0302-2838(15)00331-0.

Alkhorayef M[1], Mahmoud MZ[2], Alzimami KS[1], Sulieman A[3], Fagiri MA[4]. High-Intensity Focused Ultrasound (HIFU) in Localized Prostate Cancer Treatment. Pol J Radiol. 2015 Mar 13; 80:131–41.

Lee R, Localio AR, Armstrong K, Malkowicz SB, Schwartz JS. A meta-analysis of the performance characteristics of the free prostate-specific antigen test. *Urology* 67(4), 762–768 (2006).

Bjurlin MA[1], Meng X[1], Le Nobin J[1], Wysock JS[1], Lepor H[1], Rosenkrantz AB[2], Taneja SS[3].Optimization of prostate biopsy: the role of magnetic resonance imaging targeted biopsy in detection, localization and risk assessment. J Urol. 2014 Sep;192(3):648-58.

Murray KS[1], Bailey J[2], Zuk K[3], Lopez-Corona E[4], Thrasher JB[1,4].A prospective study of erectile function after transrectal ultrasonography-guided prostate biopsy. BJU Int. 2015 Aug;116(2):190-5

Klein EA, Cooperberg MR, Magi-Galluzzi C, et al. A 17-gene assay to predict prostate cancer aggressiveness in the context of Gleason grade heterogeneity, tumor multifocality, and biopsy undersampling. Eur Urol. 2014;66:550–560.

Cuzick J, Swanson GP, Fisher G, et al. Transatlantic Prostate Group, authors. Prognostic value of an RNA expression signature derived from cell cycle proliferation genes in patients with prostate cancer: a retrospective study. Lancet Oncol. 2011;12:245–255.

Erho N, Crisan A, Vergara IA, et al. Discovery and validation of a prostate cancer genomic classifier that predicts early metastasis following radical prostatectomy. PLoS One. 2013;8:e66855.

Mendez MH[1], Passoni NM[1], Pow-Sang J[2], Jones JS[3], Polascik TJ[1]. Comparison of Outcomes Between Preoperatively Potent Men Treated with Focal Versus Whole Gland Cryotherapy in a Matched Population. J Endourol. 2015 Jul 13.

Vu CC[1], Haas JA[2], Katz AE[3], Witten MR[2].Prostate-specific antigen bounce following stereotactic body radiation therapy for prostate cancer. Front Oncol. 2014 Jan 28;4:8.

CHAPTER 2:
Dr. William Fair Dies at 66; An Expert on Prostate Cancer ; New York Times, 2002 http://www.nytimes.com/2002/01/13/nyregion/dr-william-fair-dies-at-66-an-expert-on-prostate-cancer.html

Dr. Fair's Tumor; The New Yorker, 1998 http://jeromegroopman.com/ny-articles/DrFairTumor-102698.pdf

Li LC, Carroll PR, Dahiya R (January 2005). "Epigenetic changes in prostate cancer: implication for diagnosis and treatment." *J. Natl. Cancer Inst.* 97 (2): 103–15.

Feinberg AP. Phenotypic plasticity and the epigenetics of human disease. Nature. 2007; 447:433–40.

Boumber Y, Issa JP. *Epigenetics in cancer: what's the future? Oncology. 2011; 25:220–6, 228.*

Li LC, Carroll PR, Dahiya R (January 2005). "Epigenetic changes in prostate cancer: implication for diagnosis and treatment". *J. Natl. Cancer Inst.* **97** (2): 103–15.

Ornish, D., Weidner, G., Fair, W.R., Marlin, R., & Pettengill, E.B. (2005). Intensive lifestyle changes may affect the progression of prostate cancer. *Journal of Urology, 174(3),* 1065-1069.

Ornish D[1], Lin J, Chan JM, Epel E, Kemp C, Weidner G, Marlin R, Frenda SJ, Magbanua MJ, Daubenmier J, Estay I, Hills NK, Chainani-Wu N, Carroll PR, Blackburn EH..**Effect of comprehensive lifestyle changes on telomerase activity and telomere length in men with biopsy-proven low-risk prostate cancer: 5-year follow-up of a descriptive pilot study.** Lancet Oncol. 2013 Oct;14(11):1112-20.

CHAPTER 3:

De Lorgeril, M., Salen, P., Martin, J. L., Monjaud, I., et al., Mediterranean dietary pattern in a randomized trial: Prolonged survival and possible reduced cancer rate, Arch. Intern. Med. 1998, 158, 1181–1187.

Simopoulos, A. P., Sidossis, L. S., What is so special about the traditional diet of Greece. The scientific evidence, World Rev. Nutr. Diet. 2000, 87, 24–42.7.

Sala-Vita A. Effect of a Mediterranean diet intervention on 3T MRI-monitored carotid plaque progression and vulnerability: A substudy of the PREDIMED trial. EAS 2014; June 2, 2014; Madrid, Spain.

Mozaffarian D, Micha R, Wallace S. Effects on coronary heart disease of increasing polyunsaturated fat in place of saturated fat: a systematic review and meta-analysis of randomized controlled trials. PLoS Med 2010; 7:e1000252.

Mozaffarian D[1], Aro A, Willett WC.Health effects of trans-fatty acids: experimental and observational evidence. Eur J Clin Nutr. 2009 May; 63 Suppl 2:S5-21.

Jorge, Chavarro; Meir Stampfer, Hannia Campos, Tobias Kurth, Walter Willett and Jing Ma (2006-04-01). "A prospective study of blood trans fatty acid levels and risk of prostate cancer." *Proc. Amer. Assoc. Cancer Res.* (American Association for Cancer Research) 47 (1): 943.

Crowe, F. L., Key, T. J., Appleby, P. N., Travis, R. C., et al., Dietary fat intake and risk of prostate cancer in the European Prospective Investigation into Cancer and Nutrition, Am. J. Clin. Nutr. 2008, 87, 1405–1413.

Funk CD. Prostaglandins and leukotrienes: advances in eicosanoid biology. Science 2001;294(5548):1871–1875.

De Marzo AM, Platz EA, Sutcliffe S, et al. Inflammation in prostate carcinogenesis. Nat Rev Cancer 2007;7(4):256–269.

Demark-Wahnefried, W., Price, D. T., Polascik, T. J., Robertson, C. N. et al., Pilot study of dietary fat restriction and flaxseed supplementation in men with prostate cancer before surgery: Exploring the effects on hormonal levels, prostate-specific antigen, and histopathologic features, Urology 2001, 58, 47–52.

Augustsson K, Michaud DS, Rimm EB, Leitzmann MF, Stampfer MJ, Willet WC, Giovannucci E (2003) A prospective study of intake of fish and marine fatty acids and prostate cancer. Cancer Epidemiol Biomark Prevent 12:64–67.

Arunkumar, A., Vijayababu, M. R., Kanagaraj, P., Balasubramanian, K., et al., Growth suppressing effect of garlic compound diallyl disulfide on prostate cancer cell line (PC- 3) in vitro, Biol. Pharm. Bull. 2005, 28, 740–743.

Herman-Antosiewicz, A., Stan, S. D., Hahm, E. R., Xiao, D., Singh, S. V., Activation of a novel ataxia-telangiectasia mutated and Rad3 related/checkpoint kinase 1-dependent prometaphase checkpoint in cancer cells by diallyl trisulfide, a promising cancer chemopreventive constituent of processed garlic, Mol. Cancer Ther. 2007, 6, 1249–1261.

Hsing, A. W., Chokkalingam, A. P., Gao, Y. T., Madigan, M. P., et al., Allium vegetables and risk of prostate cancer: A population-based study, J. Natl. Cancer Inst. 2002, 94, 1648–1651.

Vasanthi HR[1], Parameswari RP. Indian spices for healthy heart - an overview. Curr Cardiol Rev. 2010 Nov;6(4):274–9.

McCann SE, et al. Intakes of selected nutrients, foods, and phytochemicals and prostate cancer risk in western New York. Nutr Cancer. 2005;53(1):33–41.

Kirsh, V.A., Peters, U., Mayne, S.T., Subar, A.F., Chatterjee, N., Johnson, C.C. & Hayes, R.B. (2007) Prospective study of fruit and vegetable intake and risk of prostate cancer. J. Natl Cancer Inst. 99, 1200–1209.

Hodge, A. M., English, D. R., McCredie, M. R., Severi, G., et al., Foods, nutrients and prostate cancer, Cancer Causes Control 2004, 15, 11–20.

Hirsh, V A. 2006. A prospective study of lycopene and tomato product intake and risk of prostate cancer. Cancer Epidemiol Biomarkers Prev, 15: 92–98.

Unlu N, et al.; Bohn, T; Clinton, SK; Schwartz, SJ (1 March 2005). Carotenoid Absorption from Salad and Salsa by Humans Is Enhanced by the Addition of Avocado or Avocado Oil. *Human Nutrition and Metabolism* 135 (3): 431–6.

Boileau, T. W., Liao, Z., Kim, S., Lemeshow, S., et al., Prostate carcinogenesis in N-methyl-N-nitrosourea (NMU)-testosterone- treated rats fed tomato powder, lycopene, or energy-restricted diets, J. Natl. Cancer Inst. 2003, 95, 1578–1586.

Johnson JJ, Bailey HH, Mukhtar H. Green tea polyphenols for prostate cancer chemoprevention: a translational perspective. Phytomedicine 2010; 17: 3–13.

Kurahashi N, Sasazuki S, Iwasaki M, Inoue M, Tsugane S. Green tea consumption and prostate cancer risk in Japanese men: a prospective study. Am J Epidemiol 2008; 167: 71–7.

Bettuzzi S, Brausi M, Rizzi F, Castagnetti G, Peracchia G, Corti A. Chemoprevention of human prostate cancer by oral administration of green tea catechins in volunteers with high-grade prostate intraepithelial neoplasia: a preliminary report from a one-year proof-of-principle study. Cancer Res 2006; 66: 1234–40.

Zhang Y, Munday R, Jobson HE, Munday CM, Lister C, Wilson P et al. (2006) Induction of GST and NQO1 in cultured bladder cells and in the urinary bladder of rats by an extract of broccoli (Brassica Italica) sprouts. J Agric Food Chem 54:9370–9376.

Singh, S. V., Srivastava, S. K., Choi, S., Lew, K. L., et al., Sulforaphane-induced cell death in human prostate cancer cells is initiated by reactive oxygen species, J. Biol. Chem. 2005, 280, 19911–19924.

Choi, S., Lew, K. L., Xiao, H., Herman-Antosiewicz, A., et al., D, L-Sulforaphane-induced cell death in human prostate cancer cells is regulated by inhibitor of apoptosis family proteins and Apaf-1, Carcinogenesis 2007, 28, 151–162.

Garikapaty, V. P., Ashok, B. T., Chen, Y. G., Mittelman, A., et al., Anticarcinogenic and antimetastatic properties of indole-3-carbinol in prostate cancer, Oncol. Rep. 2005, 13, 89–93.

Cohen, J. H., Kristal, A. R., Stanford, J. L., Fruit and vegetable intakes and prostate cancer risk, J. Natl. Cancer Inst. 2000, 92, 61–68.

Steinbrecher A, Nimptsch K, Husing A, Rohrmann S, Linseisen J. Dietary glucosinolate intake and risk of prostate cancer in the EPIC-Heidelberg cohort study. Int J Cancer 2009; 125: 2179–86.

Richman EL, Carroll PR, Chan JM.Vegetable and fruit intake after diagnosis and risk of prostate cancer progression. Int J Cancer. 2011 Aug 5.

Liu B., Mao Q., Cao M.et al; Cruciferous vegetables intake and risk of prostate cancer: a meta-analysis. Int J Cancer 2012; 19: 134–141.

Lin D.W., Neuhouser M.L., Schenk J.M., et a: Low-fat, low-glycemic load diet and gene expression in human prostate epithelium: a feasibility study of using cDNA microarrays to assess the response to dietary intervention in target tissues. Cancer Epidemiol Biomarkers Prev 2007; 16: 2150–215.

Pollak MN, Schernhammer ES, Hankinson SE. Insulin-like growth factors and neoplasia. Nat Rev Cancer 2004; 4: 505–18. lia M, Cummings JH. Physiological aspects of energy metabolism and gastrointestinal effects of carbohydrates. Eur J Clin Nutr 2007; 61 (Suppl. 1): S40–74.

Bidoli E, Talamini R, Bosetti C et al. Macronutrients, fatty acids, cholesterol and prostate cancer risk. Ann Oncol 2005; 16: 152–7.

Venkateswaran V, Haddad AQ, Fleshner NE et al. Association of diet-induced hyperinsulinemia with accelerated growth of prostate cancer (LNCaP) xenografts. J Natl Cancer Inst 2007; 99: 1793–800.

Freedland SJ, Mavropoulos J, Wang A et al. Carbohydrate restriction, prostate cancer growth, and the insulin-like growth factor axis. Prostate 2008; 68: 11–9.

Mavropoulos JC, Buschemeyer WC III, Tewari AK et al. The effects of varying dietary carbohydrate and fat content on survival in a murine LNCaP prostate cancer xenograft model. Cancer Prev Res (Phila) 2009; 2: 557–65.

Lin DW, Neuhouser ML, Schenk JM et al. Low-fat, low-glycemic load diet and gene expression in human prostate epithelium: a feasibility study of using cDNA microarrays to assess the response to dietary intervention in target tissues. Cancer Epidemiol Biomarkers Prev 2007; 16: 2150–4.

Shai I., Schwarzfuchs D., Henkin Y., et al: Weight loss with a low-carbohydrate, Mediterranean, or low-fat diet. N Engl J Med 2008; 359: 229–241.

Wright JL, Plymate SR, Porter MP, Gore JL, Lin DW, Hu E, Zeliadt SB.Hyperglycemia and prostate cancer recurrence in men treated for localized prostate cancer. Prostate Cancer Prostatic Dis. 2013 Jun;16(2):204–8.

Hong SK, Lee ST, Kim SS, Min KE, Byun SS, Cho SY et al. Significance of preoperative HbA1c level in patients with diabetes mellitus and clinically localized prostate cancer. Prostate 2009; 69: 820–826.

Hammarsten J, Hogstedt B. Hyperinsulinaemia: a prospective risk factor for lethal clinical prostate cancer. Eur J Cancer 2005; 41: 2887–2895.

Park S.Y., Murphy S.P., Wilkens L.R., et al: Fat and meat intake and prostate cancer risk: the multiethnic cohort study. Int J Cancer 2007; 121: 1339–1345.

Wallstrom P., Bjartell A., Gullberg B., et al: A prospective study on dietary fat and incidence of prostate cancer (Malmo, Sweden). Cancer Causes Control 2007; 18: 1107–1121.

Joshi AD[1], Corral R, Catsburg C, Lewinger JP, Koo J, John EM, Ingles SA, Stern MC. Red meat and poultry, cooking practices, genetic susceptibility and risk of prostate cancer: results from a multiethnic case-control study. Carcinogenesis. 2012 Nov; 33(11):2108–18.

Layton D.W., et al. (1995) Cancer risk of heterocyclic amines in cooked foods: an analysis and implications for research Carcinogenesis 16 39–52.

Joshi AD, John EM, Koo J, Ingles SA, Stern MC. Fish intake, cooking practices, and risk of prostate cancer: results from a multi-ethnic case-control study. Cancer Causes Control. 2012 Mar;23(3):405–20. doi: 10.1007/s10552-011-9889-2.

Eriksen K.T., et al. (2011) Determinants of plasma PFOA and PFOS levels among 652 Danish men *Environ. Sci. Technol* 45 8137–8143.

Chavarro JE, Stampfer MJ, Hall MN, et al. A 22-year prospective study of fish intake in relation to prostate cancer incidence and mortality. Am J Clin Nutr 2008; 88:1297–1303.

Pham TM, Fujino Y, Kubo T, et al. Fish intake and the risk of fatal prostate cancer: findings from a cohort study in Japan. Public Health Nutr 2009; 12:609–613.

Ornish D, Lin J, Daubenmier J, et al. Increased telomerase activity and comprehensive lifestyle changes: a pilot study. Lancet Oncol 2008; 9:1048–1057.

Ornish D, Magbanua MJ, Weidner G, et al. Changes in prostate gene expression in men undergoing an intensive nutrition and lifestyle intervention. Proc Natl Acad Sci USA 2008; 105:8369–8374.

CHAPTER 4:

Li Y[1], Ahmad A, Kong D, Bao B, Sarkar FH.Recent progress on nutraceutical research in prostate cancer. Cancer Metastasis Rev. 2013 Dec. 28.

Clark LC, Combs GF, Jr., Turnbull BW, et al. Effects of selenium supplementation for cancer prevention in patients with carcinoma of the skin. A randomized controlled trial. Nutritional Prevention of Cancer Study Group. JAMA 1996;276(24):1957–63.

Richie JP Jr, et al.Comparative effects of two different forms of selenium on oxidative stress biomarkers in healthy men: a randomized clinical trial. Cancer Prev Res (Phila). 2014 Aug;7(8):796–804.

Gaziano JM, Sesso HD, Christen WG, Bubes V, Smith JP, MacFadyen J, Schvartz M, Manson JE, Glynn RJ, Buring JE. Multivitamins in the prevention of cancer in men: the Physicians' Health Study II randomized controlled trial. JAMA. 2012 Nov 14;308(18):1871–80.

The effect of vitamin E and beta carotene on the incidence of lung cancer and other cancers in male smokers. The Alpha-Tocopherol, Beta Carotene Cancer Prevention Study Group. N Engl J Med. 1994;330(15):1029–1035.

Ip, C.; Birringer, M.; Block, E.; Kotrebai, M.; Tyson, J.F.; Uden, P.C.; Lisk, D.J. Chemical speciation influences comparative activity of selenium-enriched garlic and yeast in mammary cancer prevention. J. Agric. Food Chem. 2000, 48, 2062–2070.

High-SY has been found to be more effective than selenomethionine in the reducing DNA damage and an increase in epithelial cell apoptosis (natural cell death) within aging canine prostate cells. (Waters et al. 2012).

Huang HY, Appel LJ. Supplementation of diets with alpha-tocopherol reduces serum concentrations of gamma- and delta-tocopherol in humans. *J Nutr.* 2003;133(10):3137–3140.

Saldeen K, Saldeen T. Importance of tocopherols beyond alpha-tocopherol: evidence from animal and human studies. *Nutr Res.* 2005;25(10):877–889.

Jiang Q, Wong J, Fyrst H, Saba JD, Ames BN. gamma-Tocopherol or combinations of vitamin E forms induce cell death in human prostate cancer cells by interrupting sphingolipid synthesis. Proc Natl Acad Sci U S A. 2004;101(51):17825–30.

Huang Y, et al. A gamma-tocopherol-rich mixture of tocopherols maintains Nrf2 expression in prostate tumors of TRAMP mice via epigenetic inhibition of CpG methylation. J Nutr. 2012;142(5):818–23.

Wright ME, et al. Supplemental and dietary vitamin E intakes and risk of prostate cancer in a large prospective study. Cancer Epidemiol Biomarkers Prev. 2007;16(6):1128–35.

Helzlsouer KJ, Huang HY, Alberg AJ, et al. Association between alpha-tocopherol, gamma-tocopherol, selenium, and subsequent prostate cancer. *J Natl Cancer Inst.* 2000;92(24):2018–2023.

MC Myzak, P Tong, WM Dashwood, et al. (2007) Sulforaphane retards the growth of human PC-3 xenografts and inhibits HDAC activity in human subjects. Exp Biol Med 232, 227–234.

AV Singh, D Xiao, KL Lew, et al. (2004) Sulforaphane induces caspase-mediated apoptosis in cultured PC-3 human prostate cancer cells and retards growth of PC-3 xenografts in vivo. Carcinogenesis 25, 83–90.14514658.

Perocco P, Bronzetti G, Canistro D, Valgimigli L, Sapone A, Affatato A, Pedulli GF, Pozzetti L, Broccoli M, Iori R, Barillari J, Sblendorio V, Legator MS, Paolini M, Abdel-Rahman SZ. (2006). "Glucoraphanin, the bioprecursor of the widely extolled chemopreventive agent sulforaphane found in broccoli, induces phase-I xenobiotic metabolizing enzymes and increases free radical generation in rat liver." *Mutation Research* 595 (1–2): 125–136.

Singh SV, Warin R, Xiao D, Powolny AA, Stan SD, Arlotti JA *et al.* Sulforaphane inhibits prostate carcinogenesis and pulmonary metastasis in TRAMP mice in association with increased cytotoxicity of natural killer cells. Cancer Res 2009; 69: 2117–2125.

Clarke JD, Hsu A, Yu Z, Dashwood RH, Ho E. Differential effects of sulforaphane on histone deacetylases, cell cycle arrest and apoptosis in normal prostate cells versus hyperplastic and cancerous prostate cells. Mol Nutr Food Res 2011; 55: 999–1009.

Traka M, Gasper AV, Melchini A, Bacon JR, Needs PW, et al. Broccoli Consumption Interacts with GSTM1 to Perturb Oncogenic Signalling Pathways in the Prostate. *PLoS One*, 3(7): e2568.

Glinskii OV, Huxley VH, Glinsky GV, et al. Mechanical entrapment is insufficient and intercellular adhesion is essential for metastatic cell arrest in distant organs. Neoplasia. 2005 May;7(5):522–7.

Pienta KJ, Naik H, Akhtar A, et al. Inhibition of spontaneous metastasis in a rat prostate cancer model by oral administration of modified citrus pectin. J Natl Cancer Inst. 1995 Mar 1;87(5):348–53.

Eliaz I, Hotchkiss AT, Fishman ML, Rode D. The effect of modified citrus pectin on urinary excretion of toxic elements. Phytother Res. 2006 Oct;20(10):859–64.

Azemar M, Hildenbrand B, Haering B, Heim ME, Unger C. Clinical benefit in patients with advanced solid tumors treated with modified citrus pectin: a prospective pilot study. Clin Med Oncol. 2007;1:73–80.

Glinskii OV, Huxley VH, Glinsky GV, et al. Mechanical entrapment is
insufficient and intercellular adhesion is essential for metastatic cell
arrest in distant organs. Neoplasia. 2005 May;7(5):522–7.

Pienta KJ, Naik H, Akhtar A, et al. Inhibition of spontaneous metastasis
in a rat prostate cancer model by oral administration of modified
citrus pectin. J Natl Cancer Inst. 1995 Mar 1;87(5):348–53.

Guess BW, Scholz MC, Strum SB, Lam RY, Johnson HJ, Jenrich RI.
Modified citrus pectin (MCP) increases the prostatespecific antigen
doubling time in men with prostate cancer: a phase II pilot study.
Prostate Cancer Prostatic Dis. 2003;6(4):301–4.

Huang Z, Liu H. [Expression of galectin-3 in liver metastasis of colon
cancer and the inhibitory effect of modified citrus pectin]. *Nan Fang
Yi Ke Da Xue Xue Bao.* 2008;28(8):1358–1361.

Jackson CL, Dreaden TM, Theobald LK, et al. Pectin induces apoptosis
in human prostate cancer cells: correlation of apoptotic function
with pectin structure. *Glycobiology.* 2007;17(8):805–819.

Liu H, Huang Z, Yang G, Lu W, Yu N. Inhibitory effect of modified citrus pectin on liver metastases in a mouse colon cancer model. *World
J. Gastroenterol.* 2008;14(48):7386–7391.

Yan J, Katz AE. PectaSol-C Modified Citrus Pectin Induces Apoptosis
and Inhibition of Proliferation in Human and Mouse Androgen-
Dependent and -Independent Prostate Cancer Cells. *Integr Cancer
Ther.* 2010.

Azemar M, Hildenbrand B, Haering B, Heim ME, Unger C. Clinical benefit in patients with advanced solid tumors treated with modified citrus pectin: a prospective pilot study. Clin Med Oncol. 2007;1:73–80.

Eliaz I, Hotchkiss AT, Fishman ML, Rode D. The effect of modified citrus pectin on urinary excretion of toxic elements. Phytother Res. 2006 Oct;20(10):859–64.

Bemis DL, Capodice JL, Anastasiadis AG, et al.: Zyflamend, a unique herbal preparation with nonselective COX inhibitory activity, induces apoptosis of prostate cancer cells that lack COX-2 expression. Nutr Cancer 52 (2): 202–12, 2005.

Sandur SK, Ahn KS, Ichikawa H, et al.: Zyflamend, a polyherbal preparation, inhibits invasion, suppresses osteoclastogenesis, and potentiates apoptosis through down-regulation of NF-kappa B activation and NF-kappa B-regulated gene products. Nutr Cancer 57 (1): 78–87, 2007.

Yan J, Xie B, Capodice JL, et al.: Zyflamend inhibits the expression and function of androgen receptor and acts synergistically with bicalutimide to inhibit prostate cancer cell growth. Prostate 72 (3): 244–52, 2012.

Yang P, Cartwright C, Chan D, et al.: Zyflamend-mediated inhibition of human prostate cancer PC3 cell proliferation: effects on 12-LOX and Rb protein phosphorylation. Cancer Biol Ther 6 (2): 228–36, 2007.

Huang EC, Chen G, Baek SJ, et al.: Zyflamend reduces the expression of androgen receptor in a model of castrate-resistant prostate cancer. Nutr Cancer 63 (8): 1287–96, 2011.

Kim JH, Park B, Gupta SC, et al.: Zyflamend sensitizes tumor cells to TRAIL-induced apoptosis through up-regulation of death receptors and down-regulation of survival proteins: role of ROS-dependent CCAAT/enhancer-binding protein-homologous protein pathway. Antioxid Redox Signal 16 (5): 413–27, 2012.

Rafailov S, Cammack S, Stone BA, et al.: The role of Zyflamend, an herbal anti-inflammatory, as a potential chemopreventive agent against prostate cancer: a case report. Integr Cancer Ther 6 (1): 74–6, 2007.

Capodice JL, Gorroochurn P, Cammack AS, et al.: Zyflamend in men with high-grade prostatic intraepithelial neoplasia: results of a phase I clinical trial. J Soc Integr Oncol 7 (2): 43–51, 2009.

Thomas R[1], Williams M[2], Sharma H[2], Chaudry A[3], Bellamy P[4]. A double-blind, placebo-controlled randomised trial evaluating the effect of a polyphenol-rich whole food supplement on PSA progression in men with prostate cancer-the UK NCRN Pomi-T study. Prostate Cancer Prostatic Dis. 2014 Jun;17(2):180–6.

Hussain T et al. Green tea constituent epigallocatechin-3-gallate selectively inhibits COX-2 without affecting COX-1 expression in human prostate carcinoma cells. *Intl J Cancer* 2005; 113(4):660–69.

Jian L et al. Protective effect of green tea against prostate cancer: a case-control study in southeast China. *Intl J Cancer* 2004; 108(1):130–35.

Kurahashi N et al for the JPHC Study Group. Green tea consumption and prostate cancer risk in Japanese men: a prospective study. *Am J Epidemiol* 2008; 167(1): 71–77.

McLarty J et al. Tea polyphenols decrease serum levels of prostate-specific antigen, hepatocyte growth factor, and vascular endothelial growth factor in prostate cancer patients and inhibit production of hepatocyte growth factor and vascular endothelial growth factor in vitro. *Cancer Prev Res* 2009 Jun 19; online 10.1158/1940-6207.

Bettuzzi S, Brausi M, Rizzi F, et al.: Chemoprevention of human prostate cancer by oral administration of green tea catechins in volunteers with high-grade prostate intraepithelial neoplasia: a preliminary report from a one-year proof-of-principle study. Cancer Res 66 (2): 1234–40, 2006.

Brausi M, Rizzi F, Bettuzzi S: Chemoprevention of human prostate cancer by green tea catechins: two years later. A follow-up update. Eur Urol 54 (2): 472–3, 2008.

Jatoi A, Ellison N, Burch PA, et al.: A phase II trial of green tea in the treatment of patients with androgen independent metastatic prostate carcinoma. Cancer 97 (6): 1442–6, 2003.

Kaur M, Agarwal C, and Agarwal R: Anticancer and cancer chemopreventive potential of grape seed extract and other grape-based products. J Nutr 139, 1806S–1812S, 2009.

Agarwal C, Singh RP, and Agarwal R: Grape seed extract induces apoptotic death of human prostate carcinoma DU145 cells via caspases activation accompanied by dissipation of mitochondrial membrane potential and cytochrome c release. Carcinogenesis 23, 1869–1876, 2002.

Dhanalakshmi S, Agarwal R, and Agarwal C: Inhibition of NF-kappaB pathway in grape seed extract-induced apoptotic death of human prostate carcinoma DU145 cells. Int J Oncol 23, 721–727, 2003.

Raina K, Singh RP, Agarwal R, and Agarwal C: Oral grape seed extract inhibits prostate tumor growth and progression in TRAMP mice. Cancer Res 67, 5976–5982, 2007.

Singh RP, Tyagi AK, Dhanalakshmi S, Agarwal R, and Agarwal C: Grape seed extract inhibits advanced human prostate tumor growth and angiogenesis and upregulates insulin-like growth factor binding protein-3. Int J Cancer 108, 733–740, 2004.

Tyagi A, Agarwal R, and Agarwal C: Grape seed extract inhibits EGF-induced and constitutively active mitogenic signaling but activates JNK in human prostate carcinoma DU145 cells: possible role in anti-proliferation and apoptosis. Oncogene 22, 1302–1316, 2003.

Brasky TM, Kristal AR, Navarro SL, Lampe JW, Peters U, Patterson RE, White E.Specialty supplements and prostate cancer risk in the VITamins and Lifestyle (VITAL) cohort. Nutr Cancer. 2011 May;63(4):573–82.

Rettig MB, Heber D, An J et al. Pomegranate extract inhibits androgen-independent prostate cancer growth through a nuclear factor-KB-dependent mechanism. Mol Cancer Ther 2008; 7: 2662–2671.

Pantuck AJ, Leppert JT, Zomorodian N et al. Phase II study of pomegranate juice for men with rising prostate-specific antigen following surgery or radiation for prostate cancer. Clin Cancer Res 2006; 12: 4018–4026.

Jiang, J, Slivova, V, Valachovicova, T, Harvey, K and Sliva, D. 2004. Ganoderma lucidum inhibits proliferation and induces apoptosis in human prostate cancer cells PC-3. Int J Oncol, 24: 1093–1099.

Gao Y, Dai X, Chen G, Ye J, Zhou S. A randomized, placebo-controlled, multicenter study of Ganoderma lucidum (w.curt.:fr.) Lloyd (aphyllophoromycetideae) polysaccharides (ganopoly) in patients with advanced lung cancer. International Journal of Medicinal Mushrooms 2003;5(4):369–81.

Jia HQ, Wu SH, Wu J. Clinical analysis of Lingzhi spore in prostate cancer treatment. Andrology 2005;9(4):18–9.

Singh RP, Raina K, Sharma G, Agarwal R. Silibinin inhibits established prostate tumor growth, progression, invasion and metastasis, and suppresses tumor angiogenesis and epithelial-mesenchymal transition in transgenic adenocarcinoma of the mouse prostate model mice. Clin Cancer Res 2008; 14: 7773–7780.

Raina K, Rajamanickam S, Singh RP, Deep G, Chittezhath M, Agarwal R. Stage-specific inhibitory effects and associated mechanisms of silibinin on tumor progression and metastasis in transgenic adenocarcinoma of the mouse prostate model. Cancer Res 2008; 68: 6822–6830.

Terakawa N[1], Matsui Y, Satoi S, Yanagimoto H, Takahashi K, Yamamoto T, Yamao J, Takai S, Kwon AH, Kamiyama Y.Immunological effect of active hexose correlated compound (AHCC) in healthy volunteers: a double-blind, placebo-controlled trial. Nutr Cancer. 2008;60(5):643–51.

Hollis BW, Marshall DT, Savage SJ, Garrett-Mayer E, Kindy MS, Gattoni-Celli S.Vitamin D3 supplementation, low-risk prostate cancer, and health disparities. J Steroid Biochem Mol Biol. 2013 Jul;136: 233–7.

Albanes D, Mondul AM, Yu K, et al. Serum 25-hydroxy vitamin D and prostate cancer risk in a large nested case-control study. Cancer Epidemiol Biomarkers Prev. 2011;20(9):1850–1860.

Shui IM, Mucci LA, Kraft P, Tamimi RM, Lindstrom S, Penncy KL, Nimptsch K, Hollis BW, Dupre N, Platz EA, Stampfer MJ, Giovannucci E.Vitamin D-related genetic variation, plasma vitamin D, and risk of lethal prostate cancer: a prospective nested case-control study. J Natl Cancer Inst. 2012 May 2;104(9):690–9.

Aronson WJ[1], Kobayashi N, Barnard RJ, Henning S, Huang M, Jardack PM, Liu B, Gray A, Wan J, Konijeti R, Freedland SJ, Castor B, Heber D, Elashoff D, Said J, Cohen P, Galet C. Phase II prospective randomized trial of a low-fat diet with fish oil supplementation in men undergoing radical prostatectomy. Cancer Prev Res (Phila). 2011 Dec,4(12):2062–71.

Chapter 5:
Minshall C[1], Nadal J[1], Exley C[2]. Aluminium in human sweat. J Trace Elem Med Biol. 2014 Jan;28(1):87–8.

Genuis SJ[1], Birkholz D, Rodushkin I, Beesoon S.Blood, urine, and sweat (BUS) study: monitoring and elimination of bioaccumulated toxic elements. Arch Environ Contam Toxicol. 2011 Aug;61(2):344–57.

Houmard JA[1], Tanner CJ, Slentz CA, Duscha BD, McCartney JS, Kraus WE. Effect of the volume and intensity of exercise training on insulin sensitivity. J Appl Physiol (1985). 2004 Jan;96(1):101–6.

Seals DR, Hagberg JM, Hurley BF, Ehsani BF, and Holloszy JO. Effects of endurance training on glucose tolerance, and plasma lipid levels in older men and women. JAMA 252: 645–649, 1984.

Lee IM[1], Wolin KY, Freeman SE, Sattlemair J, Sesso HD.Physical activity and survival after cancer diagnosis in men. J Phys Act Health. 2014 Jan;11(1):85–90.

Kenfield SA, Stampfer MJ, Giovannucci E, Chan JM. Physical activity and survival after prostate cancer diagnosis in the health professionals follow-up study. J Clin Oncol 2011; 29: 726–32.

Richman EL, Kenfield SA, Stampfer MJ, Paciorek A, Carroll PR *et al.* Physical activity after diagnosis and risk of prostate cancer progression: data from the cancer of the prostate strategic urologic research endeavor. Cancer Res 2011; 71: 3889–95.

L.L. Ji, M.C. Gomez-Cabrera, J. Vina; Exercise and hormesis: activation of cellular antioxidant signaling pathway;Ann N Y Acad Sci, 1067 (2006), p. 425.

A.S. Fairey, K.S. Courneya, C.J. Field *et al.* Physical exercise and immune system function in cancer survivors: a comprehensive review and future directions; Cancer, 94 (2002), p. 539.

A. McTiernan; Mechanisms linking physical activity with cancer; Nat Rev Cancer, 8 (2008), p. 205.

Barnard RJ[1], Leung PS, Aronson WJ, Cohen P, Golding LA.A mechanism to explain how regular exercise might reduce the risk for clinical prostate cancer. Eur J Cancer Prev. 2007 Oct;16(5):415–21.

Jian, L., Shen, Z.J., Lee, A.H. *&* Binns, C.W. *(2005)* Moderate physical activity and prostate cancer risk: a case-control study in China. Eur. J. Epidemiol. 20, 155–160.

Shephard RJ, Shek PN. Cancer, immune function, and physical activity. Can J Appl Physiol 1995; 20: 1–25.

Lee IM, Hsieh CC, and Paffenbarger RS. Exercise intensity, and longevity in men: the Harvard Alumni Study. *JAMA* 328: 538–545, 1995.

E.L. Giovannucci, Y. Liu, M.F. Leitzmann *et al.* A prospective study of physical activity and incident and fatal prostate cancer. Arch Intern Med, 165 (2005), p. 1005.

Wiseman M. The second World Cancer Research Fund/American Institute for Cancer Research expert report. Food, nutrition, physical activity, and the prevention of cancer: a global perspective. Proc Nutr Soc. 2008;67:253–6.

Richman EL, Kenfield SA, Stampfer MJ, Paciorek A, Carroll PR *et al.* Physical activity after diagnosis and risk of prostate cancer progression: data from the cancer of the prostate strategic urologic research endeavor. Cancer Res 2011; 71: 3889–95.

Cormie P[1], Galvão DA, Spry N, Joseph D, Chee R, Taaffe DR, Chambers SK, Newton RU.Can Supervised Exercise Prevent Treatment Toxicity in Prostate Cancer Patients Initiating Androgen Deprivation Therapy: A Randomised Controlled Trial. BJU Int. 2014 Jan 27.

Cormie P, Newton RU, Taaffe DR, et al. Exercise maintains sexual activity in men undergoing androgen suppression for prostate cancer: a randomized controlled trial. Prostate Cancer Prostatic Dis. 2013 Jan 15.

Cormie P[1], Newton RU, Spry N, Joseph D, Taaffe DR, Galvão DA. Safety and efficacy of resistance exercise in prostate cancer patients with bone metastases. Prostate Cancer Prostatic Dis. 2013 Dec;16(4):328–35.

Cormie P[1], Galvão DA, Spry N, Joseph D, Taaffe DR, Newton RU. Functional benefits are sustained after a program of supervised resistance exercise in cancer patients with bone metastases: longitudinal results of a pilot study. Support Care Cancer. 2014 Jun;22(6): 1537–48.

Katzmarzyk PT, Church TS, Craig CL, Bouchard C. Sitting time and mortality from all causes, cardiovascular disease, and cancer. Med Sci Sports Exerc. 2009;41:998–1005.

George ES, Rosenkranz RR Kolt GS. Chronic disease and sitting time in middle-aged Australian males: findings from the 45 and Up Study. Int J Behav Nutr Phys Act. 2013;10:20.

Matthews CE[1], George SM, Moore SC, Bowles HR, Blair A, Park Y, Troiano RP, Hollenbeck A, Schatzkin A. Amount of time spent in sedentary behaviors and cause-specific mortality in US adults. Am J Clin Nutr. 2012 Feb;95(2):437–45.

Otten JJ, Jones KE, Littenberg B, Harvey-Berino J. Effects of television viewing reduction on energy intake and expenditure in overweight and obese adults: a randomized controlled trial. Arch Intern Med 2009;169:2109–15.

Houmard JA[1], Tanner CJ, Slentz CA, Duscha BD, McCartney JS, Kraus WE. Effect of the volume and intensity of exercise training on insulin sensitivity. J Appl Physiol (1985). 2004 Jan;96(1):101–6.

CHAPTER 6:
Carlson LE[1], Speca M, Faris P, Patel KD. One year prepost intervention follow-up of psychological, immune, endocrine and blood pressure outcomes of mindfulness-based stress reduction (MBSR) in breast and prostate cancer outpatients. Brain Behav Immun. 2007 Nov;21(8):1038–49. Epub 2007 May 22.

Cohen L, Fouladi RT, Babaian RJ, Bhadkamkar VA, Parker PA, Taylor CC, Smith MA, Gritz ER, Basen-Engquist K.Cancer worry is associated with abnormal prostate-specific antigen levels in men participating in a community screening program. Cancer Epidemiol Biomarkers Prev. 2003 Jul;12 (7):610–7.

ReicheM, Nunes SO, Morimoto HK. Stress, depression, the immune system, and cancer. Lancet Oncol. 2004 Oct;5(10):617–25. Review.

Sigurdardottir LG[1], Valdimarsdottir UA, Mucci LA, Fall K, Rider JR, Schernhammer E, Czeisler CA, Launer L, Harris T, Stampfer MJ, Gudnason V, Lockley SW.Sleep disruption among older men and risk of prostate cancer. Cancer Epidemiol Biomarkers Prev. 2013 May;22 (5):872–9.

Sigurdardottir LG[1], Valdimarsdottir UA, Mucci LA, Fall K, Rider JR, Schernhammer E, Czeisler CA, Launer L, Harris T, Stampfer MJ, Gudnason V, Lockley SW.Sleep disruption among older men and risk of prostate cancer. Cancer Epidemiol Biomarkers Prev. 2013 May;22 (5):872–9.

Kakizaki M, Inoue K, Kuriyama S, Sone T, Matsuda-Ohmori K, Nakaya N, Fukudo S, Tsuji I; Sleep duration and the risk of prostate cancer: the Ohsaki Cohort Study. Br J Cancer. 2008 Jul 8;99 (1):176–8.

Marshall NS, et al "Sleep apnea and 20-year follow-up for all-cause mortality, stroke, and cancer incidence and mortality in the Busselton Health Study Cohort" *J Clin Sleep Med* 2014;10 (4): 355–362.

Martínez-García MA, et al "Association between sleep apnea and cancer incidence: Longitudinal study of 8,900 patients from the Multicenter Spanish Cohort" *Am J Respir Crit Care Med* 185;2012: A6723.

A.S. Christensen, A. Clark, P. Salo, P. Nymann, P. Lange, E. Prescott, *et al.* Symptoms of sleep-disordered breathing and risk of cancer: a prospective cohort study. Sleep, 36 (2013), pp. 1429–1435.

Pellegrino R[1], Kavakli IH[2], Goel N[3], Cardinale CJ[4], Dinges DF[3], Kuna ST[5], Maislin G[6], Van Dongen HP[7], Tufik S[8], Hogenesch JB[9], Hakonarson H[4], Pack AI[6]. A Novel BHLHE41 Variant is Associated with Short Sleep and Resistance to Sleep Deprivation in Humans. Sleep. 2014 Aug 1;37 (8):1327–36.

Kripke DF[1], Garfinkel L, Wingard DL, Klauber MR, Marler MR.Mortality Associated With Sleep Duration and Insomnia. *Arch Gen Psychiatry.* 2002;59 (2):131–136.

Piosczyk H, Landmann N, Holz J, Feige B, Riemann D, Nissen C, Voderholzer U. Prolonged sleep under Stone Age conditions. *J Clin Sleep Med* 2014;10 (7):719–722.

CHAPTER 7:
Ho SM, Tang WY, Belmonte de Frausto J, Prins GS. Developmental exposure to estradiol and bisphenol A increases susceptibility to prostate carcinogenesis and epigenetically regulates phosphodiesterase type 4 variant 4. Cancer Res 2006; 66: 5624–32.

Murray TJ, Maffini MV, Ucci AA, Sonnenschein C, Soto AM. Induction of mammary gland ductal hyperplasias and carcinoma *in situ* following fetal bisphenol A exposure. Reprod Toxicol 2007; 23: 383–90.

Wetherill YB, Petre CE, Monk KR, Puga A, Knudsen KE. The xenoestrogen bisphenol A induces inappropriate androgen receptor activation and mitogenesis in prostatic adenocarcinoma cells. Mol Cancer Ther 2002; 1: 515–24.

Wetherill YB, Fisher NL, Staubach A, Danielsen M, de Vere White RW, *et al.* Xenoestrogen action in prostate cancer: pleiotropic effects dependent on androgen receptor status. Cancer Res 2005; 65.

Wang H, Li J, Gao Y, Xu Y, Pan Y, Tsuji I, Sun ZJ, Li XM. Xeno- oestro-gens and phyto- oestrogens are alternative ligands for the androgen receptor. Asian J Androl. 2010 Jul;12(4): 535–47.

Prins GS, Tang WY, Belmonte J, Ho SM. Developmental exposure to bisphenol A increases prostate cancer susceptibility in adult rats: epigenetic mode of action is implicated. Fertil Steril. 2008 Feb;89(2 Suppl):e41.

Kenfield SA, Stampfer MJ, Chan JM, Giovannucci E. Smoking and pros-tate cancer survival and recurrence. JAMA 2011; 305:2548–2555.

Gong Z, Agalliu I, Lin DW, et al. Cigarette smoking and prostate cancer-specific mortality following diagnosis in middle-aged men. Cancer Causes Control 2008; 19:25–31.

CHAPTER 8:

"Do Healthier Foods and Diet Patterns Cost More Than Less Healthy Options? A Systematic Review and Meta- Analysis," Mayuree Rao, Ashkan Afshin, Gitanjali Singh, Dariush Mozaffarian, *BMJ Open*, December 5, 2013.

Monsalvo et atl. 2011, Journal of Health Affairs: http://content.healthaf-fairs.org/content/30/8/1471.abstract.

Made in the USA
Middletown, DE
05 April 2019